12 Practical Steps to a New You Forever Without Arthritis

12 Practical Steps to a New You Forever Without Arthritis

"Stealing Back Your Life from Pain and Inflammation"

Authors Francisco M. Torres, MD, Board Certified
& Ashleigh Gass, MS, CSCS, CCN, CNS

Editor Abby Campbell, BSc, SFN, SSN, CPT

12 Practical Steps to a New You Forever Without Arthritis: Stealing Back Your Life from Pain and Inflammation

ISBN-13: 978-0692401781
1. Health   2. Medicine

Library of Congress Control Number: 2015935875

12 Practical Steps to a New You Forever Without Arthritis
Volume 1, First Printing May 2015, Version 1:1
(paperback edition, 5" x 8")

Authors: Francisco M. Torres, MD, Board Certified & Ashleigh Gass, MS, CSCS, CCN, CNS

Editor: Abby Campbell, BSc, SFN, SSN, CPT

For more information including quantity discounts, please visit www.ForeverYoung.MD.

Dedication

This book is dedicated to all those who are working on managing arthritis for a healthy lifestyle. Remember that your perseverance is what keeps you strong, and it is what keeps us moving steadfastly toward natural healing.

Thrive to be forever young!

Is There a Cure for Aging?

For hundreds of years, scientists and explorers have sought the fountain of youth. They've looked in remote jungles and in hidden valleys. There is an undeniable human desire to slow or ultimately stop the aging process.

Today's explorers are doctors and geneticists. They don't scour the earth and cross oceans to find what they seek. They explore in sterile labs, testing biological samples, and developing a scientific explanation for the way our bodies mature and ultimately decline.

Have they been more successful than Ponce de Leon? They have, in fact.

Scientists have discovered that we have a 125-year limit on our lifespan. We now know that each cell in our body has an "internal" clock ticking down until our time expires. This internal clock is located at the very tip of our chromosomes in a region called the *Telomere*.

When cells divide, the telomeres shorten. Unfortunately for us, Telomere length is correlated with aging and death. Therefore, the question is: *"Are the ticking clocks in our cells like time bombs we don't know how to diffuse?"*

The jury is still out to some extent. But, we do know that there are steps we can take to mitigate the shortening of our Telomeres. In fact, there are tests to measure the current length.

Once you have an idea about the length of your Telomeres, there are scientifically proven lifestyle changes you can undertake to slow the shortening process and access your internal fountain of youth. We can't live forever, but we can certainly live longer and live more abundantly.

About Dr. Torres

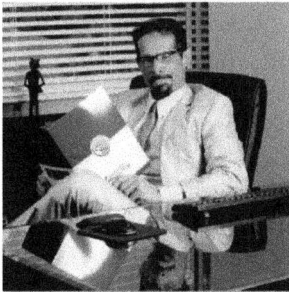

Dr. Torres specializes in the diagnosis and treatment of patients with spine-related pain syndromes and osteoarthritis of multiple joints. He has authored and co-authored several articles published in various medical journals and has also participated in several clinical research studies. His experience is vast:

- University of Puerto Rico (Cum Laude, BS Biology)
- University of Puerto Rico School of Medicine (MD)
- Veterans Administration Hospital, San Juan (Residency)
- Louisiana State University (Musculoskeletal Fellowship)
- American Academy of Physical Medicine and Rehab. (Member)
- American Association of Electro-Diagnostic Medicine (Fellow)
- International Spinal Injection Society (Member)
- American Board of Physical Medicine and Rehabilitation (Certified)
- American Board of Electro-Diagnostic Medicine (Certified)

- American Board of Pain Management (Certified)
- International Spinal Injection Society (Certificate in Discography)
- Florida Academy of Pain Management (Past Vice President)
- Osteoporosis Program of Florida Spine (Current Director)

Dr.Torres is also the President and Medical Director of ForeverYoung.MD. As a trained age-management physician, he works with patients on preventing age-related disease in order to optimize health and longevity.

About Ashleigh

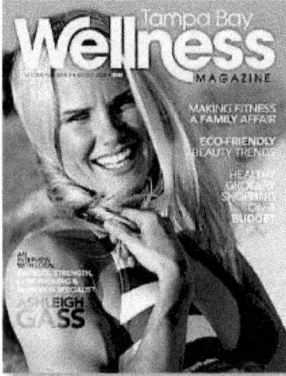

Ashleigh has been in the exercise physiology field for over 10 years. Her first degree was in Kinesiology and Exercise Physiology, from The University of Victoria, in her native town of Victoria, British Columbia, Canada. She completed her first graduate degree at The National Coaching Institute, and then her Master's degree in Clinical Nutrition from The University of Bridgeport, Connecticut. Her education is extensive and ongoing:

- Medical Exercise Specialist (MES)
- Certified Strength and Conditioning Specialist (CSCS)
- Certified Sports Nutritionist via The International Society of Sports Nutrition (CISSN)
- Certified Cross-Fit Trainer (CCFT)
- Certified Clinical Nutritionist (CCN)
- Certified Nutrition Specialist (CNS)

Ashleigh offers a host of services which include nutritional education, strength and conditioning training, and injury prevention training.

Preface

This book says it all. In the next several pages, you are going to discover a wealth of resources, skills, and tools to manage and ultimately overcome arthritis pain. I would know.

For the past twenty years, I have been a practicing rheumatologist. The treatment of different forms of arthritis is a part of my daily life. It's what I do, and I take great pride and satisfaction from the privilege of serving my patients.

I have also been an arthritis sufferer for almost as long. For nearly two decades, I have experienced pain from degenerative arthritis of the lumbar spine. Through that experience, I have come to appreciate a lot of what this comprehensive book – *12 Practical Steps to a New You Forever Without Arthritis* – makes clear in a few short pages.

Healthy choices are essential in the treatment of arthritis. Exercise, nutrition, and stress management — as this book explains — are the keys to renewed vigor.

When I injured my thoracic spine a year ago, I thought that I would not be able to exercise again. But thanks to the recommendation of my physical medicine doctor, I started doing core strengthening exercises. I experienced significant improvement in pain as well as with general muscle tone and strength. At this time, I only take medications on a limited basis and my health is better than before the injury occurred.

Arthritis has also allowed me to step back and evaluate unhealthy behaviors I had been practicing all along such as poor dieting, inconsistent exercising, and managing stress poorly. I have also seen this in my patients time and time again; those patients who become fully engaged in their treatment have the best long-term outcomes. Response to treatment is better for patients who exercise, make an effort to lose weight, and engage in healthy behaviors – rather than just expect medication to take care of all their symptoms. They come to understand that treatment of any health condition requires a holistic approach and a commitment from the patient to change or modify their lifestyle.

That is what you will find in this book. It is a synthesis of all I have learned and seen in practice, so I know it works.

In terms of osteoarthritis (the most common type of arthritis), medications are available for symptom relief – both orally and by injection. However, it is essential that patients incorporate exercise, good nutrition, and weight management as part of their treatment. In the next several pages, my fellows – Dr. Torres and Ashleigh – recommend additional options that can be incorporated to individualize treatment. Your goal of decreasing pain and improving function and quality of life for patients with osteoarthritis can be accomplished through nutritional supplements, topical remedies, and other treatments like physical therapy and acupuncture.

Rheumatoid Arthritis (RA) is another type of arthritis that can have devastating effects on overall health. RA is an autoimmune disorder where the body attacks the joints due to its systemic effects. The treatment of RA has improved dramatically over the last 15 years. Even though we cannot cure the disease, we can achieve great control of the physical manifestations – or what we call low disease activity – with early diagnosis and aggressive treatment. RA responds to prescribed medications, as directed by a rheumatologist with close monitoring of the treatment. While natural approaches – such as supplements and acupuncture – can relieve some symptoms, research is still working on a cure for RA. Because there is no cure at this time, I highly recommend – along with Dr. Torres and Ashleigh – that you be tested immediately with any suspicions that you may have RA. In addition to the joint damage RA causes, long-term inflammation increases the risk for heart disease and cancer if not treated adequately.

There are many more types of arthritis. Once the type of arthritis has been determined, a comprehensive plan needs to be organized so the patient can live and thrive with the disease. This may include the input of several specialists, and *12 Practical Steps to a New You Forever Without Arthritis* will help guide you in the planning process.

Be an effective advocate with your own physician by using the information Dr. Torres and Ashleigh have so succinctly and expertly outlined for you here. They are giving you the tools you need to effectively address the signs and symptoms of this disorder. Take an active role, stay fit, and live beyond arthritis!

Arnaldo Torres, MD, FACR

Table of Contents

"... because aging is a choice."

~ Dr. Torres

Introduction

This is not a textbook. It's not an article you can read on Wikipedia or WebMD. The next few pages are much more personal than that. You'll learn something about arthritis; that's true. But we hope that in reading this book, you learn more than just the dictionary definition. We hope you gain a holistic appreciation for what it means to live and, in fact, thrive despite the disease. This book is a practical set of suggestions, undergirded by a real passion to help all those who confront the effects of arthritis daily.

My first experience with the condition was a very personal one. My sister, Maria, had been complaining of pain in her feet and knees ever since the age of 19. After visiting a number of orthopedic specialists, she understood only that she had flat feet. The orthopedists recommended shoe inserts. It wasn't working. For over a year, she struggled through incessant pain. She could not walk from her car to her office without stopping every few yards. As we know, pain eventually leads to fear. It becomes a loss of freedom. Ultimately, that's what I witnessed developing in her.

> *"Challenges are the vehicle for growth."*

I was making my way through medical school at the time and gaining my first true understanding of how the body works. After a lecture on Rheumatic Arthritis, I called my sister and arrogantly suggested I had the answer. I was going to diagnose my first case! For some reason — likely out of desperation — Maria took her big brother's advice, and she in fact took the test. The results returned positive, and Maria finally began undergoing the proper treatment.

Just knowing the pain she felt in her joints had a name came was a huge relief. This relief, and the incremental improvement that followed, came as a jolt of confidence for me as I began my medical career. I now know better than I knew then that there is no perfect release from the pain associated with this condition. There wasn't and there still isn't for her today. But I had seen just how powerful it was for Maria to be presented with information and a plan of action. Her experience motivated me to pursue my study.

Eventually, I entered and completed a fellowship focused on the treatment of arthritis at Louisiana State University Medical School. Shortly thereafter, I was thrust into action again by another personal encounter with the disease.

I was in my first month at a new job. It was my first "real" doctor job. One of my coworkers — a woman who worked in reception — approached me for help. I recognized the look of desperation in her. It was the same look I saw in my sister when all she could do to lessen the pain was to slide ineffective inserts into the soles of her shoes. It was the look of unknowing and powerlessness.

My coworker wasn't the patient though. It turned out that her mother, living in California at the time, was suffering from extreme pain. I had felt the same sense of helplessness with my sister, so I sympathized. I asked her to have her mother come in for some tests, but she couldn't fly her out to Florida. "I can't do anything from three thousand miles away," I wanted to say. But my sister's experience encouraged me to do otherwise. I agreed to "treat" her mother over the phone.

From the onset of our call, my friend's mother detailed each of her excruciating symptoms. I felt like I was treating her just by listening. She described the parade of physicians she had been marshaled to in the past year. She lamented how not a single one of them made any difference when it came to mitigating the enormous pain she was suffering. I told her she needed to have a blood test.

> *"Make sure that those who struggle silently in our lives can feel safe asking us for help."*

I told her to focus on the sedimentation rate. I explained in the simplest terms I could that the sedimentation rate in the blood, when elevated significantly, could be consistent with a diagnosis of Polymyalgia Rheumatica. I've never heard anyone so overjoyed to learn they might have a disease. The thing is, Polymyalgia Rheumatica is treatable. You just have to know what to look for.

The woman's test came back positive and the rest, as they say, is history. The final chapter in her nearly two year battle against debilitating pain was ended with a phone call and the stroke of a pen. The proper diagnosis had made all the difference.

That's the sort of success Ashleigh and I are trying to replicate with this book. Not everyone's arthritis is treatable. There isn't any cure-all. But there are practical ways of detecting the disease in its early stages, managing its symptoms, and ultimately thriving despite its onset. We hope our message rings loud and clear, "If you have joint pain, there is hope."

Many patients walk into doctors' offices every day complaining of shoulder, hip, knee, or spinal pain. They are told after a rudimentary battery of exams that the pain they're experiencing is arthritis. Physicians begin to manage their expectations. They tell these people that arthritis will be painful and that there is no cure. They often recommend the cessation of all or most physical activity. Many patients leave these doctors' offices feeling defeated.

They buy into this approach. At the slightest inkling of pain, they stop what they're doing out of fear. Over time, disuse generates muscular atrophy. The joints don't improve. The prediction begets its own conclusion. It's a self-fulfilling prophesy.

Ash and I see these patients in our office. Once they realize that the "do nothing" approach is failing, they begin to seek solutions. They don't want to stop living. We tell them unequivocally that they don't have to.

Recovery is possible. We are passionate about making recovery a reality for all of you dealing with the signs and symptoms of arthritis. There's no need to get hooked on drugs, and joint replacement surgeries are often not the answer either. We have some suggestions. We believe in your potential.

This is not a text book. Text books are chocked full of tables and graphs and sterile sentences. The dictionary definition of a thing never truly reveals its meaning. What follows in this book is a sort of revelation. It's a reflection of the passion Ash and I feel for sharing our message of hope with all those who, like my sister and my friend's mother, were once told there was no hope. Our desire is that you find these pages enlightening and inspiring.

Warmly,

Francisco M. Torres, MD

Is Arthritis Bothering You?

Are you struggling with tenderness, swelling, stiffness, or sharp pain around your joints? Are you also dealing with other symptoms like fever, swollen glands, fatigue, weight loss, and a generalized physical discomfort? This could be arthritis.

Arthritis isn't just one disease. It's a term that actually describes more than 100 diseases that cause the symptoms you may be experiencing. Osteoarthritis is the most common form. With osteoarthritis, the cartilage around the joints wears out. Normally, this cartilage acts as a buffer between your bones. Without the buffer, bones rub together causing inflammation and pain.

We'll go over more signs and symptoms of osteoarthritis in the next few pages. Before then, we'd like to share some facts with you about this very common ailment including your risk for developing it, signs and symptoms to look out for, and how to find the right diagnosis. We'll also share conventional treatment plans before we show you 12 steps you can take to manage and relieve symptoms naturally.

How Many Have Arthritis?

Nearly 25 percent of adults (1 in 4) in the United States have been diagnosed with arthritis, an estimated 52.5 million people. Two thirds of those are under the age of 65. As the population increases, an estimated 67 million adults are expected to have arthritis symptoms by 2030.[1]

Who Gets Arthritis?

All genders, races, and ages are susceptible to arthritis. Sixty percent of those are women; 40 percent are men. Caucasians are diagnosed with the most cases at 36 million. African – Americans follow at 4.6 million and Hispanics at 2.9 million. Two-thirds of adults with arthritis are under the age of 65 with 300,000 being children under the age of 18.[2]

Additionally, nearly half (47%) of those diagnosed with arthritis haves at least one other diagnosed medical condition[3]:

- Heart disease – 47%
- High blood pressure – 44%
- Diabetes – 47%
- Obesity – 31%

Your Lifetime Risk

Whether it develops as symptomatic osteoarthritis in the knees or hips, or takes a more serious form, your risk of getting arthritis in your lifetime is nearly 50 percent. However, we can teach you what you can do to help naturally lower your risk and ultimately treat diagnosed cases.

> *"Instead of clinging to the shore, we should embrace adventure and dive deep into the ocean of possibility."*

What Type of Pain are You Experiencing?

Arthritis can be classified as *inflammatory* or *degenerative*. Inflammatory arthritis is usually referred to as rheumatoid arthritis or RA, while degenerative arthritis is best known as osteoarthritis or OA.

Causes of Rheumatoid Arthritis

Also known as an autoimmune disease, rheumatoid arthritis can be much more complicated to treat than other types of arthritis. Despite many years of intensive investigation, the cause of rheumatoid arthritis remains elusive. A number of potential culprits have been studied, including endocrine, metabolic, and nutritional factors as well as a multitude of geographical, occupational, and psychological variables. While these factors could influence the course of the disease, they clearly can't be implicated as an absolute cause for the condition.

> "Apathy is as negative as badly channeled anger."

Causes of Osteoarthritis

While osteoarthritis is known as the non-inflammatory type, inflammation may still result in the joints. However, this inflammation is a result of cartilage breakdown. Joint injury, and everyday activities that strain the joints, are the causes of osteoarthritis. This degenerative type of arthritis is usually found in the knees, hips, feet, hands, and spine.

RA and OA Similarities

Symptoms of rheumatoid arthritis and osteoarthritis are similar when it comes to stiffness and joint pain. However, the stiffness associated with rheumatoid arthritis tends to last longer than it does with osteoarthritis flare-ups. Discomfort with osteoarthritis pain is usually concentrated in the affected joint(s), while rheumatoid arthritis symptoms can include weakness and fatigue as it's a systemic disease.

Are Your Joints Simply Wearing Out?

Osteoarthritis is sometimes called degenerative joint disease or degenerative arthritis. Affecting nearly 27 million Americans, it is the most common chronic condition of the joints.[4]

With osteoarthritis, the cartilage is worn down around the joint where two ends of bones meet. With this wearing away, the bones are exposed and rub against each other. Cartilage deterioration also affects the joint's shape and makeup so that it no longer functions smoothly.

As cartilage breaks down, other problems may also affect the joint while causing irritation and pain. Surrounding tissue may be damaged, and inflammation can also occur. Potential problems include:

- cartilage and bone fragments floating in the joint fluid

- spurs or osteophytes developing

- joint fluid (hyaluronan) decreasing

You may notice trouble when walking or going up and down stairs, as these movements place stress upon the affecting joints of the back and lower body.

Osteoarthritis has no single or specific cause. Instead, several factors are involved including heredity and lifestyle. While it was once believed that the condition resulted simply from the mechanical process of "wearing out," osteoarthritis has now been declared a disease of the joint.

> *"Your attitude affects the way your story unfolds."*

Your Signs & Symptoms

Symptoms of osteoarthritis vary as it depends on which joints are affected and how severely. Some patients are debilitated while others have few symptoms in spite of dramatic joint degeneration shown on x-rays. Pain may also be intermittent where patients can be pain-free for years between symptoms.

As mentioned previously, osteoarthritis generally affects the knees, hips, feet, and lower back. When those joints are affected, difficulties ensue, even with basic daily activities such as walking, climbing stairs, and lifting objects. Neck and fingers are also commonly affected, especially the base of the thumbs. This makes grasping and holding things, such as pencils, difficult.

Stiffness and pain are usually worse in the mornings. This first movement pain usually improves during the day as daily activities are carried out. The pain may then regenerate during the evenings. Other symptoms of osteoarthritis may include:

> *"Any change has to be emotional and spiritual before it becomes physical and long-lasting."*

- warmth and swelling of one or more joints, particularly during weather changes

- localized tenderness where the joint or affected area is pressed

- steady or intermittent achy pain in the joint which is sometimes aggravated by motion

- loss of joint flexibility, such as when bending to pick up something from the floor

- crepitus which is the crunchy sound and feeling of bones rubbing together when the joint is moved

- abnormal spine curve due to imbalanced muscles from spasms

- pinching, tingling, or numbing sensations in the arms or legs

If skin turns red or feels hot, and joint pain is accompanied by a fever and/or rash, osteoarthritis is probably not the right diagnoses. If you have these symptoms, you may want to check with your healthcare provider for rheumatoid arthritis or some other possible causes.

Knees

The knee is the most common area for the development of osteoarthritis. It accounts for nearly 50 percent of all osteoarthritis diagnoses. Pain usually increases in the knee when moving and may cause warmth and swelling of the joint. As osteoarthritis increases, mobility decreases which makes walking, using stairs, and getting in and out of chairs more difficult. Sufferers may also feel or hear crepitus when moving the knees.

Hips

Osteoarthritis in the hip not only causes hip pain; it also often causes pain in the back and legs. Frequently, patients with hip osteoarthritis will have it in other joints as well. This can make it difficult to distinguish where the pain is actually originating. Failed low back decompression is the most common cause of missed diagnosis of hip osteoarthritis.

Feet, Toes, and Ankles

While each foot has 28 bones and over 30 joints, certain joints are commonly affected by osteoarthritis:

- the three foot joints involving the heel bone, inner-foot bone, and outer mid-foot bone

- the joint of the big toe and foot bone

- the joint where the ankle and shinbone meet

The ability to walk, bear weight, or even move may be affected as stiffness, swelling, tenderness, and pain increases.

Spine

Osteoarthritis of the spine is one of the most common causes of back pain. When the facet or vertebral joints become inflamed, progressive joint degeneration creates more frictional pain. In turn, back pain may progress when sitting, standing, and walking.

Neck

Osteoarthritis of the neck is also called *cervical osteoarthritis* or *cervical spondylosis*. It involves changes to the joints, bones, and discs of the neck. Neck pain and stiffness are the most common signs.

Hands and Fingers

Osteoarthritis of the hand occurs more frequently in certain areas:

- the joint at the thumb base where the thumb meets the wrist

- the joint at the end of the finger closest to the nail

- the joint in the middle of the finger

Deep, aching pain may often accompany the location at the base of the thumb which causes trouble gripping things with any kind of strength. Turning keys or opening lids may be difficult.

Symptoms over Time

As mentioned previously, osteoarthritis has different variables. For most, it usually develops over time. Some may experience achy joints only after exercise or some form of physical work with little or no pain in between. However, pain does steady over time as the cartilage between bones thin.

After long periods of inactivity, stiffness and pain may also begin to set in.

With progressive or advanced stage osteoarthritis, a single joint may be affected. However, many joints may be affected with further activity.

While it is less common, severe deformities can occur with osteoarthritis. However, it differs from inflammatory or systemic types of arthritis as it only affects joints and not the soft tissue or organs of the body as rheumatoid arthritis does. On rare occasions, osteoarthritis can lead to nerve entrapment in the spine or spinal cord of the neck.

"Being uncomfortable can be rewarding."

Finding a Diagnosis

Upon a physical examination of the affected joint(s), your doctor may order screen tests. This may include blood tests, x-rays, a magnetic resonance imaging (MRI), or arthroscopy.

Blood Tests

Blood tests are more commonly used to confirm or rule out rheumatoid arthritis. Those who have it will carry an antibody called *rheumatoid factor* or *RF*. However RF may also be present in other rheumatoid disorders. Therefore, a new test for rheumatoid arthritis may be given called *the anti-CCP test*. It is a more specific test that tends to only be elevated in patients with rheumatoid arthritis or pre-rheumatoid arthritis. The anti-CCP test can also predict how severe it may get.

X-Rays

X-rays are standard for diagnosing osteoarthritis as they can show cartilage breakdown and bone damage. However, x-rays aren't as effective for those with rheumatoid arthritis.

MRI Scans

The MRI scan can be helpful in diagnosing arthritis as it produces very clear pictures of the human body. It can reveal joint damage, especially to the spine, knee, or shoulder. Like the x-ray, an MRI can be repeated to determine the progression of the disease.

Arthroscopy

Most commonly used to diagnose knee and shoulder problems, an arthroscopy may also be used to diagnose osteoarthritis. This minor surgical procedure involves inserting a tool into the joint through several small incisions in order to detect how much joint damage has proliferated. Moreover, the doctor may repair the damage at this time. This procedure is performed on an outpatient basis.

What You Can Do for Relief

Currently, there is no cure for osteoarthritis. However, treatment can help reduce symptoms and make it possible to live an active and full life.

Treatment goals include:

- stiffness and pain reduction
- joint mobility
- damage prevention

Therapy is based on the severity of symptoms, how well other treatments have worked, and how much damage has already occurred.

Types of Conventional Therapy

Depending on the severity of your symptoms, your doctor may treat you with a program that includes any of the following:

- pain medicine, sometimes including low doses of opioids

- steroid shots

- hyaluronic acid for intra articular injections of the osteoarthritic knee

- assistive devices

- physical therapy

- occupational therapy

If your pain gets too severe, you may undergo surgery to replace the joint or keep the joints you have moving well and preventing osteoarthritis from getting worse. Some types of surgery include:

- arthroscopy

- arthrodesis

- finger or toe surgery

- osteotomy (knees and hips)

- joint replacement (knees, hips, or shoulders)

Home Treatment

Daily tasks may be difficult with arthritis, and you may not always be able to see your doctor for treatment. Other than conventional treatments, there is a variety of alternative and natural remedies you can apply to relieve stiffness and pain. We'll go over a few of these. In fact, we're going to go over 12 practical steps you can take to manage and alleviate symptoms of arthritis.

In Part I, we are going to show you how to find immediate relief for your arthritis symptoms. In Step 1, we'll teach you the appropriate times and ways to administer ice or heat to your painful joints. You'll learn the right topical creams to apply in Step 2. In Steps 3 and 4, we'll show you how to select legitimate home therapy which will help you to also discover alternative solutions to surgery.

> *"In order to succeed in life, sometimes you have to take a leap of faith and leave your comfort zone."*

In Part II, we'll help you establish transitional relief. This may take several weeks to months and sometimes years, but these methods will help alleviate pain, fatigue, and many other symptoms that often accompany arthritis. In Step 5, you'll learn the absolute best solution for relieving your symptoms. Because stress contributes greatly to the symptoms of arthritis, we'll show you how to identify your personal stress triggers and how to design a schedule for quality rest in Steps 6 and 7. We'll also show you how to manage your stress and the best ways to implement your rest schedule. Step 8 will help you identify the right shoes to wear to help you take the load off your joints.

> *"When you are guided by intuition, the world becomes a playgroun d and you enjoy a perpetual state of recess."*

Everyone diagnosed with arthritis wishes for relief. Your wishes can become a reality though if you implement each of our first eight steps. Steps 9 through 12 will help you maintain your progress and prevent further damage with specially tailored exercise routines. You'll learn how to work out and still manage your pain in Step 9. You'll boost your immunity by enjoying healing foods, supplementation, and a few old Chinese traditions in Steps 10 and 11. In our final step – Step 12 – we will show you promising new advanced treatment options that only a few specialized doctors are offering right now.

We hope you'll allow us to steal back your life from inflammation and degeneration which plagues so many arthritis sufferers. As we walk you through each of our 12 steps, be sure to engage with the step by taking action. Even if you only manage to implement a few of the steps, we are confident that you will be moving in the right direction – minimizing stiffness, aches, pains, fatigue, and other symptoms. Natural healing can assist you in overcoming symptoms without replacing them with new side effects. We hope you'll allow us to help you become a *New You Forever Without Arthritis*.

PART I: Finding Immediate Relief

✓ Using Ice & Heat Correctly

✓ Applying Creams That Work

✓ Physically Beating the Pain

✓ Discovering an Age Old Healing Art

STEP 1: Using Ice & Heat Correctly

How often throughout your childhood did your mother tell you to put ice on a "booboo?" Have you ever seen a sports movie where the athletes lounge in hot tubs or whirlpools after a game in order to relieve their aches and pains? These are basic remedies, but the proper combination of both ice and heat therapies can in fact alleviate even serous arthritis pain. So – you might ask – what is that right combination?

Discovering what works for you will take some trial and error. Eventually, however, you will learn what therapeutic measures work best to relieve your pain. Our most important piece of advice:

"Stick to it!"

Try different combinations of ice and heat therapy. It might sound a little hokey, but when you find a combination that works, keep doing it. If the pain persists, you might want to expand out into some of the other steps we describe in this book.

How Does Ice and Heat Help?

Ice and heat therapy stimulates your own body's natural healing abilities. Ice or cold compresses the sore joint and reduces swelling or inflammation by constricting blood vessels. Heat dilates the blood vessels and stimulates circulation. Heat also reduces the sensation of pain.

We'll go over ice and heat sources you can use as well as the best ways to apply both. First, we'll start with ice.

Ice Sources

When arthritis pain causes a burning sensation, it's better to apply ice or cold therapy as it can help numb the affected joint area. If your pain onset is sudden, you may also want to try ice to reduce swelling fast. Ice is also easy and cheap if your refrigerator has an icemaker at home. Any of the following will work as well:

- frozen vegetables bags

- frozen sock of rice

- frozen towel

- reusable gel-filled cold pack from your neighborhood drugstore

- local ice spray like the non-flammable fluoromethane

Best Way to Apply Ice or Cold Packs

Some of our patients prefer ice or cold therapy to moist heat therapy for arthritis pain. However, we also have patients who like to alternate sessions with both. You can experiment to see which provides you with the best relief and fits into your budget. After the onset of pain, ice or cold therapy works best when applied within 48 hours, according to the American College of Rheumatology.[5]

Cooling any areas that are red, swollen, and inflamed is important as well. Symptoms may occur from injury or overuse. In this case, elevate that body part and apply ice or cold therapy alternating for 20 minutes on and 20 minutes off.

Remember to always use a cloth or towel between your skin and the cold source. It will prevent irritation. Never leave the cold application on your skin for more than 20 minutes at a time as you don't want to allow your skin to get too cold. And, definitely remove the cold source if you notice your skin becoming blistered, bright red, blotchy, or too numb.

When Cold is Not an Option

Avoid ice or cold therapy if you have circulatory problems as it may constrict blood flow.

Heat Sources

We have noticed that patients who have ongoing pain – usually for several weeks – in a particular joint do well with heat therapy. The most effective heat therapy products are the ones that provide the appropriate temperature and are able to maintain that temperature. While warm is the proper temperature, never use a heat source that gets too hot to where it burns your skin. That will obviously only add to your discomfort. Find a tolerable temperature for showers, baths, and spas as well.

In helping our clients, we have found that the longer heat is applied, the better it is for them. For most, 15 to 20 minutes is sufficient for one session. If the pain is intense, longer sessions at 30 minutes to two hours are more beneficial.

Heat therapy can involve either moist or dry heat:

Moist Heat. Some people find that warm baths and moist heating pads provide better pain relief.

Dry Heat. While electric heating pads and saunas may draw out the body's moisture and leave skin dehydrated, some folks feel this application is better at easing their pain.

You can find many helpful heat sources in your home to use. Others may be purchased economically at your local supermarket or drugstore. Below are a few sources of heat you may want to experiment with:

- heating lamps
- heating pads (electric and moist)
- heated gel packs
- heat patches, wraps, and belts
- heated wash cloths
- hot water bottles or packs
- warm showers
- warm baths
- hot tub or whirlpool
- warm spa
- heated swimming pool
- paraffin / mineral oil mixture

Best Way to Apply Heat

As mentioned previously, you may have to experiment with different heat therapies to see which works best for you. There are a variety of ways you can apply heat for your joint discomfort. Try a few or all of them to determine which you like.

Many of our clients find that moist therapy works best. If you're stiff in the mornings, take a long warm shower after getting out of bed. The water and heat will stimulate circulation which will relieve your painful joints.

Warm baths are also very beneficial. Include Epsom salt three times per week for the most effective way to introduce magnesium into the body. The magnesium will help reduce inflammation. We recommend adding two cups of Epsom salt to your bathtub and fill with warm water (as warm as you can tolerate) and soak for 30 minutes. Many of our clients are also athletes, and we find the following bath/flexibility strategy to work well for joint repair:

- Run a bath at night, to the warmest temperature possible, using Epsom salts as described.

- Soak for 15 to 20 minutes, getting joints as warm as possible.

- Perform your specific flexibility routine (we customize this for many of our athletes).

For convenience and several hours of heat therapy, our clients have found heat patches, wraps, and belts work well.

To safely use heat therapy, make sure the temperature is never too hot as you don't want to put your skin at risk for burns. Place a cloth or towel between you and the heat source to prevent skin burns. Never apply heat longer than 20 minutes at a time or to broken or injured skin.

When Heat Is Not an Option

Please note that heat should not be applied if you suffer from the following:

- hypertension
- heart disease
- peripheral vascular disease
- deep vein thrombosis
- diabetes
- open wound
- dermatitis
- severe cognitive impairment

Additionally, swollen and bruised areas are better treated with ice or cold therapy to reduce swelling.

Summary

Ice and heat therapy are inexpensive options to provide relief from arthritic inflammation, pain, and stiffness.

STEP 2: Applying Creams That Work

Sometimes arthritis pain medication alone doesn't work. Have you ever had an especially active weekend where your joints continue to hurt even after taking your meds? Reluctant to pop another pill, you may wonder whether an over-the-counter joint cream that promises to dull that nagging pain actually works. But, will it really work? How does it work?

Topical pain analgesics or medications are formed into a cream or gel. Much like a moisturizing lotion, you would rub it over your painful joints. The ingredients are absorbed through the skin. Most people who prefer topical creams are looking to avoid the interaction of oral medications. They simply don't want to take pills or have trouble swallowing them. If this is you, a topical cream may just be the answer.

Some oral pain medications do target inflammation. The medicine travels through the bloodstream to the site of pain. However, the medicine also travels through the gastrointestinal tract, where the medicine isn't needed. Topical creams that are applied to the skin are concentrated on the surrounding pain site. While some medicines do still enter the bloodstream, the risk would be much less than it would be with oral medications.

Who Benefits Most from Topical Creams

Anti-inflammatory topical creams and gels applied to the skin work best for those with mild to moderate pain near the surface. They seem to work more for superficial joints like the hands, elbows, knees, ankles, and feet. With these areas, the medication can penetrate closer to the joint. However, we have found that topical creams don't seem to work as well for those with long-term pain that affects extended areas like the lower back, or more than one body part. Still, in most circumstances, these creams will provide some relief.

Active Ingredients of Topical Creams

The active ingredients in most over-the-counter topical pain creams may include some of the following:

Capsaicin. Capsaicin (kap-SAY-ih-sin) is the active component of several types of hot peppers which cause the burning sensation you feel when eating them. When it is used as a topical cream or ointment, it warms the skin and blocks a chemical which delivers pain messages to the brain. Examples of this cream include Arthricare, Capzasin, and Zostrix.

Salicylates and Counterirritants. Salicylates (suh-LIS-uh-lates) and counterirritants are substances such as camphor, eucalyptus oil, eugenol from cloves, menthol, oil of wintergreen, and turpentine oil. When rubbed over the joint, they produce a hot or cold sensation that temporarily overrides your ability to feel pain. Examples include AsperCreme, BenGay, Biofreeze, Flexall, Icy Hot, Myoflex, SportCreme, Therapeutic Ice, and Tiger Balm.

Topical NSAIDs. Non-steroidal anti-inflammatory drugs (NSAIDs) are commonly taken orally to relieve pain. They are better known as ibuprofen and naproxen. While there are several prescription topical creams, some are starting to become available over the counter. While oral NSAIDs seem to work better than most NSAID creams, we have found that one over-the-counter brand called Voltaren (diclofenac gel) works just as effectively when administered topically.

Your Best Choice for Topical Cream

While all the above topical creams may provide some relief, they are not all created equal. This can be very confusing – especially since some manufacturers produce several formulations with one product name, especially for creams containing salicylates and counterirritants. For example, BenGay Ultra Strength contains a whopping 30 percent salicylate while BenGay Greaseless contains a moderate 15 percent and BenGay Vanishing Cream contains no salicylate at all. Other brands, like Tiger Balm, have nearly a dozen formulations but don't list their ingredients on their labels. Then there's AsperCreme. You would think the active ingredient is aspirin, but it doesn't apply any aspirin to the skin. Talk about confusing!

Below is a table showing specific products containing salicylates and counterirritants with their percentages of their active ingredients.[6] Hopefully, this will help you decide on one or more to try.

Product	Salicylate	Camphor	Menthol
Aspercreme	10% trolamine	None	None
BenGay Greaseless	15% methyl	None	10%
BenGay Ultra Strength	30% methyl	4%	10%
BenGay Vanish. Scent	None	None	2.5%
Biofreeze	None	0.2%	3.5%
Flexall 454	None	None	7%
Flexall Maxi-mum Strength	None	None	16%
Flexall Ultra Plus	10%	3.1%	16%
Icy Hot Balm	29%	None	7.6%
Icy Hot Cream	30%	None	10%
Icy Hot Patch	None	None	5%
Icy Hot Sleeve	None	None	16%
Icy Hot Stick	30%	None	10%
Myoflex	10%	None	None
SportsCreme	10%	None	None
Thera-Gesic Maxi Strength	15%	None	1%

Because of the positive results we've seen in our clients with the NSAID cream Voltaren, it is one that we highly recommend. However, the cost is a bit more than other types of cream. Try it if your pain becomes unbearable, but give the others a shot first.

Possible Side Effects of Creams

Arthritis creams and gels are usually well tolerated. However, skin irritation may occur such as itching and redness. Sometimes, burning may occur when initially applying. Allergic reactions may also occur. Consult your doctor immediately if you have any of the following symptoms:

- hives
- lip, tongue, or face swelling
- breathing difficulties
- closed throat

Summary

While over-the-counter topical creams are a viable choice in relieving arthritis pain, please remember that some ingredients still enter your bloodstream. Be sure to use only as directed by the packaging or by your personal physician.

STEP 3: Physically Beating the Pain

Like many people with arthritis, you probably experience days from time to time in which the pain is especially difficult to manage. One way of fighting it is through a soothing massage. There's just a calming effect on the stress and tension of constant pain that can be rewarding.

Whether conducted in a beautiful day spa or a physical therapy clinic, massage is something many people use to soothe sore joints and muscles. It can even help you relieve anxiety and sleep better, both of which are typical concerns associated with the pain. Recent research has even shown massages can affect the body's production of certain hormones linked to blood pressure, heart rate, and other key vital signs.

Many wonder if massages are effective for only the anxiety and stress that sometimes occurs from arthritis pain? Some have been skeptical about whether or not the treatment can actually help alleviate the root cause of the pain.

Regular massage of joints and muscles can lead to pain reduction in people with arthritis. This simple therapy can improve stiffness, pain, range of motion, handgrip strength, walking, and overall joint function. A recent study showed consistent and regular massage therapy over an 8-week period significantly improved in all areas for people with arthritis compared to those who didn't undergo therapy.[7] Another study reported that massage reduced lower back pain significantly in those diagnosed, and the benefits lasted at least six months.[8] In our own clinic, we have seen pain relief with nearly all of our clients who have undergone massage therapy.

The level of pressure used in massage is what matters most for people with arthritis. A 2010 study published in the *International Journal of Neuroscience* reported that stimulating pressure receptors or nerves under the skin conveys pain-reducing signals to the brain with moderate pressure.[9] While light pressure can be stimulating, it only touches the surface of the skin superficially. Moderate pressure is the key.

How Massage Therapy Works

If you've ever had a massage, whether at a spa or at home, you know that it can relieve both physical and mental stress. Massage lowers the production of the stress hormone called cortisol, and it also boosts the *feel good* hormones called serotonin. It can also lower production of a chemical in the brain called a neurotransmitter that is often linked with pain. While there are many variables involved with how massage works to ease symptoms of arthritis, the actual mechanism is still under investigation. Clinical studies and testimonies of those with arthritis just know it works.

Types of Massage Therapy

Depending on the type of massage, therapy can be soothing or rough and intense. Different techniques and healing philosophies fall under the massage umbrella. In general, massage is the manipulation of the body's muscles and connective tissues. Your therapist may use his or her own hands, but mechanical tools may also be applied to the body's surface. Sometimes massage therapists employ cold and heat applications, as well as lotions or oils. You may obtain a massage from a trained and licensed therapist, or you can massage your own joints and muscles. Below are a few types of massage therapy. You may want to try different ones, or even combinations of a few, to find out which is right for you.

Anma. This Japanese massage involves kneading of the muscles and other soft tissues with no oils. Anma is based on the philosophy that energy flow in the body is disrupted, and practitioners believe that massage can restore this flow, activating the body's natural ability to heal itself.

Ayurvedic Massage. As a natural health philosophy, Ayurveda blends massage, yoga, meditation, and herbs. Ayurvedic massage, also known as *abhyanga*, is a full-body massage using aromatic oil for purported spiritual healing.

Deep Tissue Massage. Deep tissue massage often requires intense and focused pressure on the manipulation of both the top and deeper muscle and tissue layers. Oils are typically used as well. Massage is designed to address severe tension and pain. It may cause lingering soreness which may not be appropriate for everyone with arthritis.

Hot Stone Massage. With hot stone massage, smooth heated stones are placed on your back as you lie on your stomach. The hot stones heat the muscles and tissues to release tension and promote relaxation. Therapists will also knead your muscles by hand in addition to placing stones on the skin.

Lomi Lomi. This Hawaiian therapy is considered a healing practice that may involve diet, prayer, meditation, and other healing techniques in addition to massage of the muscles and tissues.

Myofascial Release. Myofascial release involves manipulating the fascia and connective tissue surrounding muscles, blood vessels, and nerves in order to relieve pain. Your therapist will stretch and release those connective tissues by gently rolling the skin back and forth. Usually no oils are used when performing this type of massage therapy.

Reflexology. As an alternative Asian healing practice, reflexology is based on the belief that pressure of particular areas on the body, such as the hands and feet, will spur healing. It is meant to promote pain relief, as well as reduce anxiety and stress.

Rolfing. Similar to myofascial release, Rolfing is part of a healing philosophy called *structural integration*. It involves the therapist moving the body into certain positions and manipulating fascia tissues. It aims to promote pain relief and relaxation, as well as restore posture and range of motion.

Self-Massage. You can massage your own joints, pressure points, or muscles by using your hands, knuckles, elbows, or massage tools. You may also use mechanical tools to offer heat or vibration, as well as household objects like tennis balls, to reach areas such as your back. Self-massage works especially well for relieving stiffness and pain in hands, arms, knees, calves, feet, and neck.

Shiatsu. Widely performed in the United States, shiatsu is actually a Japanese massage technique. Fingers and palms are used in a continuous and rhythmic motion on specific points along the body. Shiatsu is also a healing philosophy thought to restore healthy energy in the body. No oils are used, and you usually remain completed clothed during the session.

Swedish Massage. As the most common type of massage, Swedish massage involves long and fluid strokes to the muscles and tissues to reduce stiffness and aches in the muscles and joints, as well as reduce anxiety. Lotion or oil is typically used with five basic strokes: effleurage (sliding or guiding of hands across skin), petrissage (muscle kneading), tapotement (rhythmic knuckle tapping against the skin), friction (moving across fibers), and vibration or shaking of the body. Pressure may be adjusted according to your stiffness and pain.

Thai Massage. Placing the body in yoga-like positions, as well as using more flexibility stretching, Thai massage applies pressure to the muscles and joints.

Trigger Point Massage. By applying pressure or vibration into myofascial trigger points, this type of massage is designed to relieve pain in specific areas of the body. Trigger points are areas in the body that may have formed knots, and the pinpointed pressure is designed to relax those knots and muscles.

Caution Using Massage Therapy

If you have the slightest worry about the use of massage therapy, it would be a good idea to get a thumb's up or down from your physician. It's also very important to let your massage therapist know if you are uncomfortable or having pain with the techniques being used. Your therapist will appreciate the feedback. While therapists can usually tell if you have inflammation in a particular area, always be sure to let him or her know that you have arthritis before the first session. Massage should never increase your anxiety, stress, or pain. If it hurts, be sure to let your therapist know or discontinue therapy.

Summary

Your goals for massage therapy may vary. Whether you are interested in relieving anxiety and stress caused by arthritis, or you are seeking relief from the stiffness, be sure to talk with your massage therapist about your goals. This will help your therapist plan sessions with the appropriate techniques.

STEP 4: Discovering an Age Old Healing Art

It's been 2,500 years in the making, but this age old healing art is becoming more mainstream. Research has proven that acupuncture can relieve and heal the symptoms of both rheumatoid arthritis and osteoarthritis. On the ground, it has provided relief to many of our clients. Ultimately, it may be an option for you to try as well. But before you seek out acupuncture treatment, you should understand a little about the theory behind the practice first.

Both ancient and modern-day acupuncture are both based on something called *qi* which is pronounced "chee." Qi is considered an essential life energy that flows within the body alongside 20 invisible channels known as *meridians*. When the flow of this energy is out of balance or blocked, pain and illness occur. Connected to the meridians are 2,000 acupuncture points. By stimulating these points with needles, the flow can be corrected and then alleviate pain.

However, current research has now proven the scientific efficacy of acupuncture as well. While it was traditionally used to prevent, diagnose, and treat disease, it is now considered a complete medical protocol focused on correcting energy imbalances within the body.

How Acupuncture Works

In acupuncture therapy, thin needles are inserted into the skin. This technique stimulates specific acupuncture points to correct imbalances within the body. To help you understand, imagine cutting your hand. Your body is like the sounding alarm alerting the need for emergency care, so it naturally sends help to fight the battle with clotting factors for healing. With acupuncture, the body pays special attention and sends healing to the micro-trauma from needles inserted to the acupuncture points. These points usually surround painful joints with those who have arthritis, and this ancient healing art releases the pain. It can also stimulate the release of your natural pain fighters called *endorphins* which help regulate your body's nervous system.

In addition to treating chronic degenerative diseases such as arthritis, acupuncture is used to treat many conditions that contribute to physical and emotional pain:

- neurological problems (migraines and Parkinson's disease)

- digestive complaints (nausea, vomiting, irritable bowel syndrome)

- respiratory conditions (sinusitis and asthma)

- gynecologic disorders and infertility

- emotional disorders (anxiety and depression)

- addictions

- fatigue

Types of Acupuncture

Although acupuncture originated in China, it has spread throughout the world – from Japan, Korea, and Vietnam to Europe and the Americas. Based on differing opinions about theory and technique, many styles have developed over the centuries. However, there is no evidence that one style is more effective than another. While there are now many styles, American doctors use acupuncture for treating and managing pain in their patients. Following are two of the most popular styles:

Traditional Chinese Acupuncture (TCM). No matter what your condition may be, TCM's focus is to promote balance within the body. When the body is balanced, the theory is that your entire being will function optimally, while balancing your physical, mental, emotional, and spiritual being. TCM is the most common form of acupuncture practiced in the United States.

Electroacupuncture. Similar to traditional acupuncture, electroacupuncture uses the same points in the body for stimulation during treatment. Just like TCM, needles are used. However, in electroacupuncture therapy, the needles are attached to electrical impulse devices. The devices can be controlled to adjust the intensity and frequency of the impulses being delivered. Electroacupuncture only uses two needles at a time so that the electrical current can pass from one needle to the other. Several needle pairs can be simultaneously stimulated but no longer than 30 minutes at a time. The advantage of using electroacupuncture, compared to more traditional forms of acupuncture, is that the insertion of needles does not need to be precise as the electrical current delivers to a larger area. Another advantage is that electrodes can be used instead of needles for those who have a fear of needles.

Treatment Outcome

Rheumatoid Arthritis

Both TCM and electroacupuncture have been shown to reduce tenderness in people with rheumatoid arthritis. A Chinese study in recent years performed 20 sessions throughout a 10-week period using both styles of acupuncture on patients between the ages of 48 to 68 who had been diagnosed with arthritis for 2.5 years to 15.5 years. Pain was significantly reduced.[10]

Osteoarthritis

Acupuncture of osteoarthritis has also shown positive results. A significant 2006 German study evaluated 304,674 patients who were in the care of more than 10,000 physicians and received 15 sessions of acupuncture for chronic osteoarthritis pain of the hip or knee, low back pain, neck pain, or headache. Treatments were given over a period of three months. The study found that acupuncture, in addition to standard medical care, is an effective treatment and can last for three months after the last session.[11]

Acupuncture Risks

The risks of acupuncture are low, especially when working with a licensed acupuncture practitioner. In rare cases, there may be minor bleeding or bruising with both traditional and electroacupuncture due to needles being injected into small blood vessels. With electroacupuncture, you may feel a tingling sensation due to the electrical current but most people do not experience any pain. People who should avoid electroacupuncture are those with:

- a history of seizures, epilepsy, heart disease, and stroke

- a pacemaker

- a bleeding disorder or taking blood thinning medication

Areas of the body that electroacupuncture should avoid:

- head
- throat
- directly over the heart

Electrical currents should also never travel across the midline of the body which extends from the bridge of the nose to the bellybutton.

If you are considering electroacupuncture, be sure to talk to you doctor about its potential risks and benefits. If you are pregnant, also speak with your doctor as some types of acupuncture may stimulate labor. Finally, make sure your acupuncturist is licensed and always use sterile, disposable needles.

Summary

Many of our clients use acupuncture as a measure for pain management and healing, along with their regular age management treatments. You may also find relief from this protocol.

PART II: Establishing Transition Relief

✓ *Finding Ways to Manage Weight*

✓ *Calming Stress Triggers*

✓ *Scheduling Enough Sleep & Rest*

✓ *Slipping in Shoe Relief*

STEP 5: Finding Ways to Manage Weight

You may already know that maintaining a healthy weight is beneficial for your overall health. However, if you're like most people, achieving a healthy weight can be challenging. Still, even a few pounds lost can relieve arthritis symptoms. *(If you're currently at a healthy weight and have a good body mass index, you may skip this step.)*

According to the Centers for Disease Control and Prevention, 69 percent of American adults over the age of 20 are considered overweight. Half of those overweight are obese.[12] Weight is attributed to medical conditions like heart disease, diabetes, arthritis, and more. However, health problems (including arthritis) can be reduced with weight loss. A modest reduction of five or 10 pounds can offer meaningful health benefits for those who are overweight or obese, even if they never achieve their *ideal* weight.[13]

Benefits of Weight Loss

Let's take a look at some benefits of weight loss for arthritis conditions:

Joint Pressure Reduction. A study in *Arthritis & Rheumatism* found that one pound lost can relieve as much as four pounds of pressure from the knees.[14] If you can lose just 10 pounds, that's 40 pounds of pressure removed.

Pain and Inflammation Ease. A couple of clinical studies have indicated that weight loss lessens pain, lowers inflammation, and improves overall function.[15] Exercise can manage and lessen symptoms of arthritis as well.[16]

Weight Loss Challenges

If you've been on the path of losing weight but having difficulties, you're not alone. Our clients declare the scale gets stuck all the time. The most surprising things can keep you from trimming down and losing unwanted pounds. We've highlighted a few of the most difficult diet challenges, as well as solutions, below. However, we'll discuss what you can do to supercharge your weight loss in a healthy and correct way in Part III.

Diet Soda and Artificial Sweeteners. The largest sources of calories in the American diet include regular soft drinks. Therefore, many people opt for *diet* sodas. However, they may not realize that even diet soft drinks contribute to weight gain. In fact, one diet soda per day can increase your weight by a whopping 41 percent and put you at risk for obesity.[17] For those who drank two or more diet drinks for 10 years, the risk of obesity increased to 500 percent! How so? It seems that diet sodas contain a chemical that cause sugar cravings and increase appetite.[18]

> **Solution:** Swap your diet soda for water or herbal tea. If you can't live without your diet soda, try cutting back to no more than one every other day. After two weeks, cut back to every third day. Continue cutting out a day of sodas every two weeks until they are no longer part of your diet. For coffee and tea, try using pure Stevia in place of your artificial sweeteners like NutraSweet, Equal, Sweet-n-Low, and Splenda. Native to South America, Stevia is an herb that has no calories yet tastes much sweeter than table sugar. Stevia also contains nutritive properties that are good for your body as

well – vitamin B3, potassium, zinc, and magnesium.

Healthy Restaurants. Many diners bill themselves as *healthy*. However, believing in this misconception can backfire your weight loss efforts. You may end up eating more calories at restaurants that display a healthy image (think Subway) than the traditional fast-food joints like McDonalds.

> **Solution:** Before you dine at a restaurant, do your homework. Visit the restaurant's website to look over its menu's nutrition information. Choose an entrée that contains less than 500 calories with a healthy portion of protein such as lean beef, chicken, turkey, fish, or seafood. If you don't have the opportunity to check out the restaurant's menu before arriving, ask them for their menu's nutrition facts. Every restaurant should have one. Also, many entrées come loaded with starchy carbs like French fries, mashed potatoes, or rice. Toss them aside or limit them to only a few bites.

Free Days. Many diet programs allow a *free* day to keep your dieting from being too restrictive. However, this is not an effective strategy as most people tend to overeat and make poor food choices on their free days. In fact, a study by the National Weight Control Registry found that people who cheated on their diets during the weekends and holidays actually regained their weight after one year.[19]

>**Solution:** Create a little *wiggle* room in your daily calorie count. By allowing 150 bonus calories each day, you can still satisfy cravings if need be, yet you won't blow your healthy eating habits.

How to Lose Weight

As you now know, weight loss can literally take a load off your joints. The connection between weight loss and pain relief for people with arthritis can be huge. You may also know that diet and exercise are part of the weight loss equation. However, there is a right way for using weight loss protocols, especially for arthritis. We will uncover several ways in future chapters.

Summary

While weight loss challenges do affect the majority of the population, you can use the strategies provided in this chapter as well as some of our practical steps in Part III. By applying our solutions, you can lose weight effectively which will help you relieve arthritis pressure and pain.

STEP 6: Calming Stress Triggers

Some periods of our lives are smooth sailing. Without the stress, our body's organs, and the chemicals produced from them, are in balance. However, living in this *Utopia* is not an everyday reality for most of us. Whether it's personal, financial, or work related – or a combination of some or all – stress can spin us out of control like cars on a slick highway. Under normal stress, your hormones can put you back on track and headed down the road again. Within moments, they can help you navigate through life again whether it is lifting a bad mood, breaking a fever, or reducing pain.

While our bodies are intelligent and know just how to produce enough hormones to protect us from physical or emotional stress, excessive stress can wreak havoc on your chemical messengers which, in turn, cause other chemical messengers to fail to do their jobs efficiently. Heart rate, blood pressure, body temperature, metabolism, sleep, pain perception, immune system response, and appetite can all be affected. Joint pain and inflammation may even occur.

Stress Management Techniques

Although stress can take its toll on you, you can decrease its damaging effects by practicing methods to reduce it. Finding the right strategy is the key. You may find taking a walk in the country works well for you, while your best friend may find a hot bubble bath in candlelight works better. Just knowing you have the power to control your disease with strategies to reduce stress is a stress reducer in itself. Our clients have found some of the following Mindfulness-Based Stress Reduction (MBSR) techniques to calm their stress triggers. You may also find they work for you as well.

Focus and Breathe. Two techniques you may use to manage stress are *Diaphragmatic Breathing (DB)* and *Progressive Skeletal Muscle Relaxation (PSMR)*. In DB, consciously inhale deeply through your nose and exhale through your mouth at the same time you are expanding your diaphragm. With PSMR, visualize a word, phrase, or image that you feel is relaxing. With your entire body – from head to toes – tighten, hold for a few seconds, and then release groups of muscles one at a time. You may want to start from the top of your body and move down towards your toes, or vice versa. With this technique, do several sets until you are relaxed.

Release Negativity. Another MBSR technique can help you release negative or self-defeating thoughts by releasing your negative thoughts and helping you into relaxation. For those who can't sleep, this technique works especially well. Also, become aware of any self-defeating thoughts. As we acquire pain and grow older, stress ignites with thoughts like "I'm too young to have pain" or "I'm getting old." To try this technique, get into a comfortable position and close your eyes. As the negative or self-defeating thought comes to you, imagine it drifting off like a cloud or sailing down a stream until you can no longer see it.

Keep a Journal. You can reduce stress and release any negative emotions like anger and anxiety by keeping a daily journal. A study conducted by the Southern Methodist University found that people feel a purpose and make positive life changes when they spend 20 minutes writing in a journal about their emotional circumstances.[20]

Exercise. When stress starts to build, a short brisk walk or meditative exercise such as yoga can relieve stress. One study published in the *Annals of Behavioral Medicine* suggests 90 minutes of yoga reduces perceived stress and cortisol levels.[21] We have seen many of our clients start yoga with much frustration. However, their flexibility increased and their stress and pain dramatically decreased. With a little determination, you too can find benefits through yoga. Try meditative or relaxing types of yoga like Hatha, Vinyasa, Iyengar, or Restorative.

Summary

Not all stress is avoidable. However, you can take steps in managing the triggers that are within your control. By doing so, your body will be more balanced and will ease the pain that comes with arthritis.

STEP 7: Scheduling Enough Sleep & Rest

Are you dreaming of sleep only to be roused by pain several times each night? If you are, you are not alone. Arthritis may be a major cause. Constantly readjusting your pillow can become an arduous chore. The problem may seem intractable, but there are ways to improve your chances of getting a truly good night's rest. We've seen some of the following tips help many of our clients. They could very well help you deal with arthritis-related sleep trouble as well.

How Much Sleep You Need

According to the National Sleep Foundation, you need approximately seven to 9 hours of sleep each night.[22] Older adults (65+) may need only seven to 8 hours, and children may need more. Ideally, sleep comes in cycles of 90-minute segments throughout those hours. It includes rapid eye movement (REM) sleep which is considered your *dream* stage, but you first enter four other stages. Each stage takes you to a deeper and more restorative stage until you enter that wondrous REM sleep. After the cycle is complete, you resurface and enter another 90-minute segment. These cycles continues throughout the night until you awaken.

Insomnia Symptoms

Sometimes, you may have a disruption of your sleep cycle. If it becomes a habitual disruption where you become restless and can't sleep, you have insomnia. Insomnia is common among adults, but it's usually very temporary. Many of us experience short-term insomnia lasting less than three months. Chronic insomnia lasts more than three months with at least three episodes each week.[23]

Common symptoms of insomnia may include:

- fatigue
- lack of focus or concentration
- poor memory
- mood disturbance
- sleepiness during the day
- low energy or motivation
- increased accidents or errors

Arthritis' Contribution to Insomnia

Insomnia comes in two forms. There is no clear cause for why people can't sleep when they have *primary* insomnia. Researchers are still investigating this phenomenon. However, *secondary* insomnia is a side effect of certain conditions like arthritis. It can be caused by stress, worry, pain, medications, as well as poor sleep hygiene. Normal aging can also cause insomnia. As you get older though, you still need sleep even if your body makes it more difficult.

The Pain and Sleep Disruption Cycle

Chronic arthritis pain can be a huge discomfort to your sleep. According to Luis F. Buenaver, Ph.D., an assistant professor of psychiatry and behavioral sciences at Johns Hopkins University School of Medicine, approximately

80 percent of people with chronic pain experience disturbances in their sleep.[24]

Clinical studies have also shown that people are more sensitive to pain when they are awakened by it. This may be due to the impacts of sleep deprivation on inflammation, pain, and the immune system.[25] Buenaver has something to say about this:

> "Such pain catastrophizing has been found to be a more robust predictor of worse pain and pain-related disability than depression, anxiety, and neuroticism."

In other words, that nagging pain may be disrupting your sleep cycle where you never complete the four stages or REM before starting over again. However, your psyche may also be contributing to your insomnia.

Your pain and your psyche both contribute to the seemingly endless cycle of sleep disruption. The more you don't sleep, the worse pain you feel. The more pain you feel, the worse your sleep disruption. It can be a vicious cycle wreaking havoc on your body and your brain.

The Sleep Cycle and Memory Connection

For people with Alzheimer's and dementia, sleep is extremely important. Brain chemicals called neurotransmitters are important as they help your body recharge while you sleep. They help improve your memory. If properly recharged, they help you remember what you've learned, heard, or seen while you were awake. Some of these neurotransmitters peak during REM sleep; therefore, it's important to go through the entire 90-minute sleep cycle.

How You Can Get More Rest

As we mentioned earlier, sleep disturbances can be caused by stress, worry, pain, medications, and poor sleep hygiene. Below, we will go over a few techniques that may help alleviate each of these triggers. However, you may have to experiment with each technique to find the right solution for your insomnia.

Relieve Stress and Worry

Stress and worry can cause pain as your cortisol levels rise. We like to ask our clients if they have any control over the things they are stressing about. Usually, they tell us they don't. So, why do it? All you can do is your best at whatever it may be, so just relax. Try some of the following techniques to help you relieve stress:

- **Relax your face.** Tighten all your facial muscles and hold for two seconds. Take a deep breath. Relax muscles while exhaling. Repeat a few times.

- **Buy a memory foam pillow.** You can purchase memory foam pillows for your neck, your back, and your hip. Once you've found the most comfortable position, you don't have to fight with your pillow each night.

- **Space your fitness routine.** Spread your exercises out instead of cramming your weight training, cardio, and other exercises into one session. Never overextend yourself.

- **Meditate.** Visualize your worries and imagine them being carried off downstream until they disappear over the horizon. Continue doing this with all your worries until you are just relaxing near a soft flowing stream. Listen to the flow of water and the birds singing. Smell the nearby flowers, and feel the warm sun shining down on you. Relax.

- **Take a hot bubble bath.** A soothing hot bath before bedtime may relax you.

Reduce Pain

Try a few or all of the other steps we have included in this booklet for relieving pain naturally.

Modify Medication Schedules

Because arthritis medications can cause sleep complications, you may need to modify the way you take them, including the dosage and times. Corticosteroids, prescribed for joint inflammation, may cause you to be alert and awake. On the other hand, painkillers (including NSAIDs) may cause sleepiness and make you want to nap during the day. Talk to your doctor about taking your anti-inflammatory pain medication during the day and your narcotic pain relievers at night. Also, try other remedies to accommodate your pain during the day so you won't be tempted to nap.

Alter Poor Sleep Hygiene

By changing a few simple habits, you can improve your sleep routine greatly. Try a consistent schedule for going to bed and waking up. In the hours before bedtime, try relaxing activities. Turn off any electronic devices like your phone, computers, and televisions as they disrupt your circadian rhythm. Change into comfortable clothing. Try a relaxing yoga, meditation, or a hot bubble bath. Avoid caffeine and sugar after morning hours, and drink an herbal tea made for relaxation and sleep before bedtime. If you're napping during the day, cut that time in half or try not to nap. You may be surprised at how well you sleep just by changing a few of these habits.

Summary

There is hope when it comes to overcoming secondary insomnia. Stress and worry are major contributors. Be consistent with your sleep, practice intentional relaxation techniques, and be mindful of your medication schedules.

STEP 8: Slipping in Shoe Relief

If your feet hurt from arthritis pain, it's difficult to think much about anything else. Even everyday activities like standing or walking can be a daunting task. Improvising your stance or position to relieve the pain can also cause pain for your ankle, knee, hip, and back. Who wants that?

This problem, it turns out, is quite common. One in four adults suffers from foot pain. By redistributing weight, orthotics or specially made shoes can relieve pressure on your foot's sensitive areas, as well as improve foot function. In fact, orthotics can provide cushioning that reduces stress or biomechanical load to your lower body, while correcting gait and structural abnormalities.[26] However, one must understand the biomechanics and alignment of the lower extremity to effectively treat arthritis of the foot and ankle. Gait analysis and a thorough examination of the foot and shoe are essential before treatment with orthotics. If the examination can predict how the foot will function during weight bearing, then the correct orthotics can be prescribed or recommended.

Slowing Arthritis Progression

According to a Cochrane Review, the right inserts or shoes may also help slow the progression of arthritis.[27] Several studies have found compelling evidence to support the proposition that specially-made orthotics are able to reduce foot pain in people with rheumatoid arthritis, juvenile idiopathic arthritis, and plantar fasciitis or osteoarthritis-related heel pain.

More research needs to be done to figure out specific benefits such as how long someone may need to wear orthotics before feeling better and if there are lasting benefits after disuse. However, current evidence proves that orthotics do relieve pain. According to Dr. Jim Christina, director of Scientific Affairs for the American Podiatric Medical Association, 80 to 85 percent of patients who use custom-fit orthotics get symptom relief.[28] Another study showed that the semi-flexible type of orthotic device to be the most useful and the best accepted device available. The major disadvantage was its limited durability. Almost 80 percent of the 235 patients evaluated in the study experienced 50 percent improvement in their symptoms.[29]

Where to Buy Orthotics

Your doctor can determine whether you would be a good candidate for orthotics. He or she can refer you to a podiatrist who can examine your feet, ankles, knees, and hips. The podiatrist will also observe and evaluate your gait. If you need orthotics, these providers can recommend options for you which can be over-the-counter or custom orthotics.

The Cost of Orthotics

Your cost for a pair of custom orthotics may range between $300 and $800. Some medical insurance plans may cover a portion or all of the cost depending on your diagnosis. The upfront cost of orthotics may seem a little hefty at first, but you'll get several years of wear with your orthotics – usually 3 to 5. The cost also includes moldings for your feet.

More economical over-the-counter orthotics may suit you as well. They usually don't last as long as the custom-fit orthotics because they are made of softer materials. However, they can provide some relief if you can find a pair that suits you. Over-the-counter inserts range from $10 to $80.

Over-the-Counter Orthotics

Although the efficacy of custom orthotics is backed by scientific research demonstrating symptom relief in 80 to 85 percent of users, not everyone will want to opt for the more expensive route. You can still find over-the-counter orthotics if you know where to look. Many of our clients have found relief from the following:

Athletic Shoes

Our clients frequently tell us that their feet feel best wearing athletic shoes. By wearing athletic shoes, much of the pressure they feel in their foot and ankle joints is relieved. This is interesting because our clients have only confirmed what a clinical study reported in the *Journal of Bone and Joint Surgery*. In fact, the study showed that training shoes reduced the impact pressure in the forefoot by 60 percent and the inner soles by 17 percent.[30] Nike, Reebok, and other well-known brands provide custom-fit training shoes. Ask your sales representative at your favorite sports performance store or check them out online.

Dr. Scholl's Custom Fit® Orthotic Inserts

Some of our clients have received great relief with Dr. Scholl's Custom Fit® Orthotic Inserts. You can have your feet analyzed at one of Dr. Scholl's kiosks in your local drugstore. These kiosks use FootMapping® technology to gather measurements for your feet. Once measured, this free self-service then recommends the right inserts for you. The cost of Dr. Scholl's Custom Fit® orthotics is approximately $50.

REI's SOLE Thin Sport Custom Footbeds

Our clients have also raved about REI's SOLE Thin Sport Custom Footbeds as they are better than the straight over-the-counter orthotics. In fact, they are more like custom-fit orthotics. But, REI's is an over-the-counter brand providing moldable inserts. To find the right fit, all you have to do is heat the molds in your oven for two minutes. Then put them into your shoes and stand in them for two minutes without moving. While REI's inserts are better than the straight over-the-counter version, you need to ensure the moldable inserts are properly placed within your shoes in order to get a good impression and fit. Our athletic clients find REI's inserts work well for skiing, hiking, and running as they balance moisture and friction.

Other Over-the-Counter Orthotics

Many over-the-counter inserts are made from soft materials that only last for a short time. If you decide to try over-the-counter orthotics, just make sure you find one with a plastic polymer or a hard plastic that's a little more rigid than just the typical shoe insole.

Summary

Custom or over-the-counter orthotics may provide you with a ton of arthritis pain relief if you are having problems with your feet, ankles, knees, hips, or back.

PART III: Enjoying Lifelong Relief

- ✓ Exercising with Arthritis
- ✓ Eating to Reduce Inflammation
- ✓ Fighting Pain with Supplements
- ✓ Exploring Upcoming Modern Medicine

STEP 9: *Exercising with Arthritis*

Many people with arthritis joint pain choose to (and are sometimes told to) "stop doing what hurts." Unfortunately, this can include most activities. Due to pain and fear of making their symptoms worse, our new clients often tell us they have quit their fitness endeavors, as well as other activities like walking, playing with children, and doing simple household chores. They become sedentary, bored, and depressed. Muscle atrophy, obesity, and increased joint dysfunction begin to plague them. Needless to say, ceasing all activities can be more crippling than even the symptoms of arthritis.

Arthritis shouldn't represent a permanent barrier to exercise or being active. It's your body's way of saying:

> *"Hey! You have way too much pressure and friction in this joint! You had better fix this problem or arthritis will keep grinding down your joints!"*

If you address the mechanical failures that produce pressure and dysfunction on your joints, you will experience relief; you will allow yourself to become productive again without constant pain. To fix your problems, you need a good team on your side. That includes a physician who will help you understand why you have arthritis and encourage you to take action through movement. You will also need a good physical therapist, as well as a knowledgeable exercise trainer. Both should be familiar with arthritis so they can help you rehabilitate your body, especially the symptomatic joint(s) of arthritis. Your team will work together with you to form goals to set goals such as:

- preserving or restoring range of motion and flexibility around the affected joint(s)
- increasing muscle strength

- improving endurance through aerobic conditioning

While many doctors believe the best treatment for arthritis is to stop moving the symptomatic joint, we believe that symptomatic joints, as well as surrounding muscles, need *movement* for the best relief. Our belief also coincides with numerous clinical studies. In fact, the Johns Hopkins Arthritis Center advises[31]:

> *"Physical activity is essential to optimizing both physical and mental health and can play a vital role in the management of arthritis. Regular physical activity can keep the muscles around the affected joints strong, decrease bone loss and may help control joint swelling and pain. Regular physical activity replenishes lubrication to the cartilage of the joint and reduces stiffness and pain. Exercise also helps to enhance energy and stamina by decreasing fatigue and improving sleep. Exercise can enhance weight loss and promote long-term weight management in those with arthritis who are overweight."*

Exercise Readiness Assessment

Let's face it. Habits are difficult to break or to make. Sometimes, understanding that you need to adjust your habits is hard to contemplate. Therefore, your exercise trainer should assess whether you are in fact ready to start an exercise program. Your psychological readiness is just as important as your physical readiness as it will help you stick with a program and succeed. Both your doctor and your exercise trainer need to address self-awareness and goals.

If you are ready and willing to be more active, your doctor will go over your medical history and conduct a physical exam. An evaluation, which may include X-rays and CT scans, will assess the severity of your affected joint(s), as well as the surrounding joints, muscles, and tissues. Your doctor will then refer you to a physical therapist who specializes in arthritis. He or she will work with you to determine where the patterns of dysfunction originate and help you rehabilitate those areas.

You can complete further training with a certified strength and conditioning specialist or exercise trainer who is knowledgeable about arthritis. Before designing your individual plan, your trainer must test you. The American College of Sports Medicine recommends the following exercise testing program for individuals with arthritis[32]:

- muscle strength and endurance
- aerobic endurance
- joint flexibility and range of motion

- neuromuscular fitness, including gait analysis and need for orthotics
- functional capacity to accomplish activities of daily living

Beginning a Correct Exercise Regimen

An expert will be able to develop an exercise training program for arthritis based on your personal need. For this, you will have to advocate on your own behalf. The program must be based on the arthritic joint(s) involved, as well as the extent of the damage. Following are a few approaches to exercise you may find helpful to keep in mind:

Structured Exercise Programs. Your physical exercise trainer can build a structured exercise program to help you with strength, mobility, and flexibility. This may include weight training, as well as a form of exercise that includes aerobic conditioning. The largest clinical trial to evaluate the effects of exercise on osteoarthritis – The Fitness Arthritis and Seniors Trial (FAST) – reported that both resistance training and aerobic exercise three times per week for 40 minutes each session showed significant improvements in symptoms of physical disability, performance, and pain.[33]

Range of Motion & Flexibility Programs. You may have a limited range of motion with arthritis, especially in your lower back, hips, and knees. If so, your loss of function places you at risk for injury and falls. Many doctors will advise stretching. This advice is actually not specific enough. Affected arthritic joints may be lax and already overstretched which can make you more vulnerable to injury. An optimal daily exercise plan is needed to maintain cartilage health which should include range of motion exercises. Regular compression and decompression is necessary for the cartilage surrounded by the affected joint(s) to stimulate remodeling and repair.[34]

Water Aerobics. One of the best exercise regimens for arthritis is aquatic aerobics, especially when training occurs in therapeutic pools where the water temperatures are usually warmer than recreational pools (e.g., 78-83 degrees Fahrenheit). Most therapeutic pools also have ramps which make it easy to enter and exit the pool for exercise. In a large clinical study, aerobic conditioning with water aerobics showed significant improvements in aerobic capacity, walking time, depression, anxiety, and physical activity after 12 weeks of training. Range of motion was more greatly improved in participants of aquatic aerobics than in those who did nonaerobic training for range of motion.[35]

Recreational or Lifestyle Exercise. To achieve health benefits, physical activity does not need to be strenuous. According to the Surgeon General, moderate amounts of physical activity can be obtained in longer sessions or in accumulating shorter sessions which is also recommended for older adults.[36] Leisure, occupational, or household activities are all considered *lifestyle activities* that are at least moderate in intensity. Examples include walking, raking leaves, and gardening. For people with arthritis, lifestyle physical activity may be very appropriate. If you've been sedentary, short durations of moderate intensity exercise, as opposed to a longer continuous session, may reduce pain and prevent injury. Intermittent sessions also provide individuals with arthritis rest in between exercise sessions.

Adapting to Exercise

The American Council of Sports Medicine has outlined several exercise modifications for people with arthritis[37]:

Begin slowly and progress gradually. People with arthritis often have lower levels of fitness due to stiffness, pain, and biomechanical abnormalities. During a flare, too much exercise may result in increased inflammation, pain, and damage to the joint(s). Therefore, a gradual progression is the goal for movement complexity, intensity, and duration. Alternating activity with rest should be the initial goal.

Avoid rapid or repetitive movements. You should emphasize joint protection strategies if you suffer from arthritis. Avoid repetitive movements that are highly percussive in nature. Exercise speed should match biomechanical status, and you should place special attention on joints that are misaligned and unstable. For instance, fast walking speeds increase stress on the joints. Therefore, walking speed should match your biomechanical status so more damage does not occur.

Match physical activity to your needs. Swelling, stiffness, pain, and structure changes may restrict your range of motion and cause your arthritic joint(s) to be unstable. Therefore, extra care should be taken to prevent further damage. Adapting physical activity to your needs is important.

Summary

By retraining the affected arthritic area – both from a muscular and neural perspective – you may benefit from:

1. the removal of joint inflammation
2. increased hydration and nutrition to the joints

Continuing exercise and physical activity will help minimize your symptoms of arthritis. We have seen it with our own clients, and we encourage you to continue as well. Having several exercise options and locations provides you with alternatives on days you can't get out of the house. It also keeps you from becoming bored.

STEP 10: Eating to Reduce Inflammation

Inflammation is the cornerstone of the body's healing response. It provides extra nourishment and opens avenues for renewed immune activity to the site of injury or infection. When you injure your hand or knee, you can see inflammation at work in swelling and redness. You can also feel the heat and pain.

However, inflammation can sometimes persist or serve no purpose. From it, your body can become sick and damaged such as in the case of arthritis. Studies have shown that sustained inflammation also induces degeneration of the joints.[38/39]

Therefore, prevention and improving symptoms are important. Nutrition is a key factor in managing inflammation because what you eat can affect your joints when they are under stress or wear-and-tear from exercise, labor intensive jobs, or just moving constantly.

How Diet Can Make or Break Your Joints

Clinical studies have demonstrated that joint degeneration is worsened by high sugar, low-fat, low-protein, and pro-inflammatory diets.[40] Some foods that belong to these categories include breads, muffins, cereals, dried fruit, frozen dinners, and more. If you're filling your belly with these so-called foods, you'll most likely pay a hefty price long-term.

If you're eating poorly every day, your body just isn't getting properly fed with the right vitamins, minerals, phytonutrients, and fatty acids to protect it from the brutal attacks of inflammation. With chronic inflammation, joint cartilage is more susceptible to wear and tear. In addition, your own immune system may get mixed messages and begin attacking what it's supposed to protect.

How to Eat to Reduce Inflammation

We've already discussed some of the foods that may be causing you to suffer the painful symptoms of arthritis. But, fear not! Treating your arthritis by correcting your diet does not mean eating like a sad rabbit. An anti-inflammatory diet is actually chocked full of yummy alternatives to pain-producing foods. We'll go over these with you.

Other than the right foods, we'll also go over the best supplements and herbs to combat arthritis in the next chapter. A well-rounded nutrition plan combines nutrient-dense foods, supplements, and herbs. We bet you'll be surprised at what you can actually eat. Better yet, you'll be surprised at how great you feel. After reading Steps 10 and 11, make a plan to clean out your refrigerator and pantry. Go shopping and stock up on joint-friendly foods.

As mentioned earlier, chronic inflammation is usually a source of arthritis. While inflammation is normal and beneficial when your body is fighting bacterial and viral invaders, it leads to trouble when it begins to run out of control. Diet is usually the culprit for causing inflammation in your body to "go rogue."

There are a number of foods that contain anti-inflammatory properties, so make sure you include them in your diet. Below are eight of the most powerful foods for relieving or preventing pain from arthritis.

Cold-Water Fish

Animal-based Omega-3 fatty acids can be found in cold-water fish such as wild Alaskan salmon, tuna, mackerel, herring, sardines, and anchovies. In addition to fighting inflammation, diets rich in these fish can reduce inflammation and oxidative stress.[41]

Regular intake of cold-water fish has been found to reduce the incidence of inflammatory diseases such as arthritis. Pick a few of your favorite cold-water fish and include it in your diet at least three times per week.

Coconut Oil

You may have heard of coconut oil's miraculous benefits in recent years. Research has shown it to be an extremely valuable source for many health conditions, including arthritis, due to its antioxidant and anti-inflammatory action. In a recent experimental study, coconut oil was used to treat arthritis.[42] The results demonstrated less edema formation and cellular infiltration upon supplementation. Many of our clients have reaped many beneficiary effects from using coconut oil. Include it in your diet, especially when cooking as it holds up to high heat much better than olive oil. You may also find it in supplementation form.

Extra Virgin Olive Oil

One of the healthiest diets in the world is the *Mediterranean Diet*. It includes a relatively high consumption of dietary fat, mostly extra virgin olive oil which is a monounsaturated fatty acid. The beneficial effect of olive oil has been widely studied and could be due to the phytochemicals it contains which also include anti-inflammatory properties. A recent study published in *The Journal of Nutritional Biochemistry* confirmed the importance of including olive oil in the diet when exercising.[43] Together, olive oil and exercise help to prevent osteoarthritis disease as it "preserves the articular cartilage and then the entire joint." Instead of eating processed salad dressings, make a point to include extra virgin olive oil as a dressing along with red wine vinegar. You may also add it to your cooked vegetables as a flavor enhancer.

Vegetables and Fruits

You can obtain important sources of nutrients, dietary fiber, and phytochemicals from vegetables and fruits.[44] They all contain antioxidants, flavonoids, carotenoids, and vitamin C, which all protect against cellular damage. Dark leafy green veggies such as spinach, kale, and collard greens contain exceptionally powerful nutrients which help to reduce inflammation. Cruciferous vegetables like broccoli, cauliflower, and Brussels sprouts are also important as inflammation mediators.[45] Include a wide range of vegetables and fruits as a staple in your diet to reduce arthritic inflammation. A decent goal is 10 servings per day. One serving includes a half cup cooked or one cup raw vegetables. A sample fruit serving is one-half of a small apple, pear, or banana. Blueberries and raspberries are powerful antioxidants, so one-fourth of a cup is a serving.

Fermented Veggies

An optimal gut flora boosts immunity and helps ward off chronic inflammation. Fermented foods such as sauerkraut and kimchi will help reseed beneficial probiotic microbes in your gut. Fermented veggies are a rich source of probiotics and are capable of restoring gastrointestinal barrier integrity and down regulating inflammation in the gut specifically.[46]

Mushrooms

While some may be poisonous, others contain strong compounds that discourage inflammation.[47] Mushrooms provide prebiotic factors to support beneficial probiotic microbes. They also provide a complex nutritional matrix of vitamins, chelated minerals, enzymes, proteins, and amino acids. While shiitake mushrooms can be easily found in your local market, you may also want to try the following when you can find them: reishi, antrodia, cordyceps, king trumpet, and lion's mane.

Garlic

For centuries, garlic has been treasured for its medicinal properties. It's also one of the most heavily researched plant foods with over 170 studies proving its benefits for more than 150 conditions. Garlic's benefits include antioxidant, anti-bacterial, anti-viral, and anti-fungal properties. Its therapeutic effects are thought to come from its sulfur-containing compounds, allicin, which eradicates the most dangerous free radicals more effectively than any other known compound.[48] Add it to your veggies and marinades for its powerful benefits as well as to flavor your foods.

Berries

Compared to most other fruits, berries rate very high in antioxidant capacity. Blueberries, raspberries, and blackberries are also low in sugar. Berries contain polyphenol compounds purported to have anti-inflammatory activity.[49] The most notable polyphenols in berries are anthocyanins which are responsible for the beautiful colors of these fruit.

Herbal Teas

Green tea, specifically Matcha, is nutrient dense and has up to 17 times the antioxidants of wild blueberries.[50] Not only that, the concentration of a polyphephenol called *epigallocatechin gallate* (EGCG for short) is 137 times greater than China Green Tips green tea and at least three times higher than the largest literature value of other green teas.[51] EGCG is a potent anti-inflammatory, as well as an antioxidant, anti-viral, and anti-carcinogen. Tulsi is another tea loaded with anti-inflammatory compounds that support immune function. Turmeric and ginger teas are also well-known for reducing the inflammatory response.

Summary

Eating an anti-inflammatory diet is one of the best things you can do to reduce pain in your body. Remember to eat wholesome foods that are full of nutrients. Cold-water fish, vegetables, and fruits are known to heal the body. For a natural medicinal boost, try sauerkraut, kimchi, mushrooms, garlic, berries, and herbal teas.

STEP 11: Fighting Pain with Supplements

Dozens of supplements are billed as being effective at combatting the symptoms of arthritis. Not all have been thoroughly tested though. It is true that *some* supplements have been empirically proven to be more effective at combatting arthritis than prescription medications. But the science can be tricky. Minimal results might occur in people who haven't traded out their processed diets for nutrient-dense ones. For those of you who take our advice on food seriously, supplements can in fact be quite effective. Below are just a few you might want to try.

All supplements and herbal remedies have been tested and shown to work. However, you may want to consult with your physician prior to taking any supplement, especially if you are on any prescription medication. When trying a new supplement, only try one at a time for a few weeks. This will help you determine where side effects are coming from if they should occur.

Boswellia Serrata

Also known as *Indian Frankincense*, Boswellia Serrata is an herbal extract taken from a tree with the same name. Resin made from the extract has been used for centuries in Asian Ayurvedic and African folk medicine to treat several health conditions, including chronic inflammatory illnesses such as rheumatoid arthritis and osteoarthritis. Boswellia Serrata has also been proven to be an effective pain killer. Evidence proves that this herbal remedy provides the potential benefits in recovering articular cartilage damage and protection from degradation due to inflammation.[52] The standard dose is 300 to 400 milligrams three times per day.

Chondroitin & Glucosamine

New clinical trials report that chondroitin and glucosamine sulfates are beneficial for osteoarthritic knee joint pain and function. The supplement increases a type of collagen which is able to reduce inflammation and cellular death. In turn, it is also able to improve the anabolic and catabolic balance of the extracellular cartilage matrix.[53] The improved balance may also help regenerate the affected joint structure(s), leading to reduced pain and increased mobility.[54] Daily dosage depends on your weight. If you are less than 100 pounds, take 800 milligrams of chondroitin with 1,000 milligrams of glucosamine. If you weigh more than 100 pounds, take 1,200 milligrams of chondroitin and 1,500 of glucosamine.

Gamma Linolenic Acid

In a Cochrane review of herbal therapies for rheumatoid arthritis, gamma linolenic acid (GLA) in primrose oil, borage seed oil, and black currant seed oil proved beneficial. Evidence included reduced pain and improved disability.[55] Take two to three grams in divided dosages daily. Make sure that whatever oil you take carries the appropriate amount of GLA. You may find any of the oils in capsule or liquid form.

Ginger

Since ancient times, Asia has used ginger medicinally to *bring warmth*. Part of anthroposophic nursing, ginger therapy has been used to manage chronic inflammatory conditions such as osteoarthritis. In a typical case study, ginger therapy activated remarkable relief of symptoms which progressively improved over 24 weeks.[56] Ginger comes in capsules, tinctures, teas, powder, oils, and food. Capsules are usually the purest form, and you may try 100 to 200 milligrams daily for four to six weeks. If you take a blood-thinning medication, like warfarin (Coumadin), do not take ginger as it may reverse the effects of the medication.

Glucosamine & Omega-3

Research also shows that glucosamine taken with Omega-3 may be stronger when taken together.[57] According to researcher Joerg Gruenwald, Ph.D., "Omega-3 fatty acids inhibit the inflammation process in osteoarthritis, whereas glucosamine sulfate further supports the rebuilding of lost cartilage substance."

Green-Lipped Mussel Extract

Green-lipped mussel is a shellfish from New Zealand. It has shown promise in relieving osteoarthritis pain of the hips and knees. In a clinical study, patients reported a 53 percent reduction in pain relief. After 8 weeks, they reported 80 percent pain relief and better joint function.[58] Another study in 2013 reported green-lipped mussel showed significant improvement in patients compared to patients who took fish oil. The group that took green-lipped mussel reported an 89 percent decrease in pain symptoms, and 91 percent of the patients reported an improved quality of life.[59] Take 1,150 to 1,500 milligrams per day in divided doses of the stabilized extract or 900 to 1,380 milligrams per day of the freeze-dried preparation.

Hyaluronic Acid

This naturally occurring polymer is found in every tissue of the body and is concentrated particularly in the skin and synovial fluid. However, it decreases with age. According to a study published in *The Scientific World Journal*, oral administration of polymer hyaluronic acid alleviates osteoarthritis symptoms when combined with exercise.[60] Research shows 200 milligrams of hyaluronic acid is a reasonable daily dosage in capsule form.

Omega-3 Fish Oil

As mentioned in the previous section, Omega-3 fatty acids are helpful in reducing inflammation and oxidative stress. A study at Brigham and Women's Hospital in Boston also revealed that Omega-3s actually convert compounds that are 10,000 times more potent than the original fatty acids themselves.[61] These compounds help bring inflammatory response in the body to an end. Take 2.6 grams twice daily.

Pine Bark Extract

In a large clinical study, 100 patients were treated for three months using either pine bark extract (also known as *Pycnogenol*) or a placebo for treating symptoms of osteoarthritis. Results showed the extract improved symptoms in patients with mild to moderate osteoarthritis. Improvements were so great that they no longer needed non-steroidal anti-inflammatory drugs (NSAIDs) such as ibuprofen or naproxen.[62]

Turmeric/Curcumin

While turmeric has been used for centuries as an Ayurvedic medicine for inflammatory disorders, modern studies now back up what we already knew. In fact, a 2006 study showed turmeric to be even more effective in *preventing* joint inflammation than reducing it.[63] Another clinical trial found that turmeric supplementation provided long-term improvement in pain and function in 100 percent of patients.[64] A pilot study in 2012 showed that curcumin, the most active constituent of turmeric, reduced joint pain and swelling in rheumatoid arthritis patients better than non-steroidal anti-inflammatory drugs (NSAIDs).[65]

Summary

Supplements have been proven effective for treating arthritis symptoms. Before opting for an invasive treatment protocol, you may want to try one of the supplements we have listed.

STEP 12: Exploring Upcoming Modern Medicine

To date, current treatment options for arthritis are limited to pain reduction and joint replacement surgery. We've presented you with many options for preventing, improving, and sometimes healing arthritis. We would now like to share some information on developing modern medicines. Specifically, we'll go over three types of treatments currently being studied in the scientific community that have proven successful for people who cannot find relief from their pain and other symptoms:

1. Prolotherapy
2. Stem Cell Regeneration Therapy
3. Platelet Rich Plasma Therapy

All three of these new treatments provide hope for people with severe arthritis.

Prolotherapy

Advanced medical therapies can also protect you from severe arthritis and its associated pain and disability. One such therapy is Regenerative Injection Therapy or RIT, otherwise known as Prolotherapy or Sclerotherapy. It was named RIT by Doctor Felix Linetsky in 1999 because scientific observation of the technique had revealed that tissue proliferation happened only for a short period of time, but regeneration and repair can persist much longer.[66]

RIT was actually described over 130 years ago.[67] It was described in somewhat different terms, but the benefits of this therapy were fundamentally understood even then. It effectively repairs injured or degenerated connective tissues, like ligaments, tendons, or cartilage – all involved in causing your joints to hurt.

The therapy involves injections into these connective tissues.[68] These injections introduce either (1) chemical agents or (2) biological agents into the affected area. The result tracks the natural healing processes of these structures. Every joint relies on the proper function of the connective tissues. Arthritis pain is often caused by a failure of these very tissues.

Chemical Agents

Chemical agents can include concentrations of Lidocaine (a local anesthetic you might be familiar with from your last cavity filling or cleaning at the dentist) combined with dextrose (sugar) and other irritating ingredients like phenol or glycerin to get the connective tissues going. A 2012 study published in *Pain Medicine* demonstrated the effectiveness of the Lidocaine and Dextrose injections that lasted for more than 24 weeks after 32 weeks of therapy for knee osteoarthritis. In combination with exercise, participants showed a 36.2 to 47.3 percent improvement.[69] Another study on athletes indicated a 78 to 82 percent improvement in pain with no returns to therapy.[70]

Biological Agents

In the second group are the biological agents PRP (Platelet Rich Plasma) or PPP (Platelet Poor Plasma), chorionic fluid, and chorionic membrane derived from stem cells, adipose stem cells, or fat cells obtained from the patient's own bellies, or bone marrow stem cells also obtained from the patient herself.

There's no scientific consensus about which of these options is better. Based on our own observations, the authors currently prefer PRP, PPP, or the chorionic fluid and membrane from stem cells.

RIT Outcome

A series of RIT injections over time should yield improved strength and eventually lead to normal function of the joints involved, with its associated pain relief. RIT is potentially valuable wherever there is persistent pain and tenderness around ligaments or tendons. Pain from larger joints, like shoulders, knees or hips, as well as from small spinal joints, can all be treated with RIT. In fact, recent advances in ultrasound allow for precise RIT injections in any portion of tendons affected with the degenerative process called tendinosis.

Stem Cell Regeneration Therapy

For treating disease and replacing or regenerating diseased tissue, stem cells have tremendous potential. To fully understand what a stem cell is and how it works may be a little more complicated than this book allows. In a nutshell, stem cells differ from other types of cells within the body. They start off unspecialized yet are capable of renewing themselves through cell division. Sometimes, they may be inactive for a long period of time. However, they may become specialized as they serve to repair or replenish other cells that are worn out or damaged. Stem cells usually come from two main sources – embryos and adult tissue.

Embryonic Stem Cells

Embryonic stem cells are derived from human embryos that are four or five days old. They are usually extracted from extra embryos created during in-vitro fertilization. They are the most potent since they must become every cell type within the body. For instance, embryonic cells continuously divide and generate specialized cells that make up your tissues and organs.

Adult Stem Cells

Adult stem cells (also called *somatic stem cells*) exist throughout the body after embryonic development. They are found inside different types of tissues such as the brain, bone marrow, blood, blood vessels, skeletal muscles, skin, and liver. These stem cells remain dormant for years until they are activated by tissue injury or disease. They are able to divide and renew by themselves indefinitely, and they are able to generate a range of cell types from the original organ or even regenerate the entire organ. Evidence has also proved that adult stem cells have the ability to specialize into other cell types.

Tissue and Organ Regeneration

With stem cell regeneration therapy, more people can be helped and sometimes saved from death. Currently, donated organs can be transplanted to help someone in demand for that organ. However, the demand far exceeds the supply. Unfortunately, many patients must wait for someone to die in order to receive a donated organ. However, stem cells can potentially be used to grow a particular type of tissue or organ.

In the case of arthritis, 2015 shows promise for stem cell regeneration therapy. By demonstrating anti-arthritic effects, the anticipation is that stem cells implanted in arthritic cartilage will treat osteoarthritis by producing tissue to heal the cartilage defect.[71/72] Studies have also been very promising for people with rheumatoid arthritis and other autoimmune inflammatory diseases.[73/74/75]

Platelet Rich Plasma Therapy

Another innovative, new therapy is also underway to treat osteoarthritis. *Platelet Rich Plasma* or *PRP* is being used to treat inflammation and pain, as well as slow the progression of osteoarthritis. It may also be able to stimulate cartilage regeneration. The earlier the disease is treated, the more effective the therapy is as it slows the progression of arthritis.

How PRP Works to Relieve and Heal

In the natural healing process, your body sends platelet cells in the bloodstream to the maligned site. Because platelets are packed with healing factors, they initiate the repair process and attract critical help from stem cells. PRP has the potential to fill cartilage defects to enhance cartilage repair, improve joint function, and reduce symptoms.[76]

PRP therapy intensifies the natural healing process as it delivers a higher concentration of the platelets into the connective tissue. To create PRP, a small sample of your blood is drawn and placed in a machine called a *centrifuge* which spins the blood at high speeds and separates the platelets from the other components of blood. This concentrated PRP is then injected back into the site of injury. It's a jumpstart to healing naturally.

Recent studies in 2015 have proven PRP to be an effective treatment for osteoarthritis and more efficacious than hyaluronic acid treatment.[77] PRP therapy with therapeutic exercise can be even more effective in pain reduction and stiffness compared to exercise alone.[78]

Summary

With advances in medicine, and promising clinical studies, hope is only a step away from reality. For people who have not found relief from natural remedies or traditional medicines, you will soon be saying your *good-byes* to arthritis.

Our Personal Note to You

✓ The Best Remedy for a "Bad Back" by Francisco M. Torres, MD

✓ Overcoming Pain with Healthy Practices by Ashleigh Gass

The Best Remedy for a "Bad Back"

"So, you have a bad back, do you?"

Get up and move! It's not as big a problem as you think....

Over a decade ago, I was diagnosed with a "bad back." My doctor took X-rays and an MRI of my lower spine. The picture below is a current X-ray and an MRI of my lower back which is not much different from the one he looked at 10 years ago – maybe somewhat better. When he showed the results to me, he insinuated that I was doomed. That sounds extreme, but many people hear the same thing from their own doctors. I thought the days of strenuous physical activity, or even running long distances, were a thing of the past.

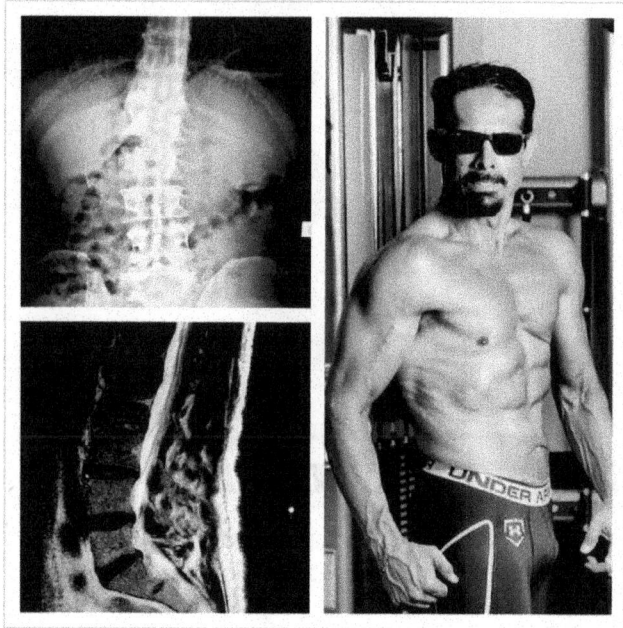

Since that diagnosis, I've completed several half marathons, as well as an Ultra Marathon. I've even won first place in bodybuilding competitions. That wouldn't have been possible without strenuous strength training. I continue to be active with TRX® Suspension Training which is a form of exercise that develops strength, balance, flexibility, and core stability simultaneously. It is a program developed by the United States Navy Seals. Additionally, I have continued with long distance running. My bad back hasn't stopped me yet! I'm happy to say that the *expert* doctor who insinuated I would be doomed was wrong.

Eight out of ten Americans will feel back pain during the course of their lives. Unfortunately, back pain is the second most common reason for visits to the doctor. Pharmacy shelves are stocked to the brim with expensive back braces and pulls, pain potions, and other gimmicky cures. Can we even count the number of television commercials for *special* beds to help your back?

Back pain has been touted as a mysterious, long-term condition that needs special devices, strange exercise plans, and medicines or surgery for pain and symptom relief. The worst thing about back pain is that doctors tell their patients that they must give up their favorite activities and accept pain as a routine part of life.

From there, the cycle begins!

Back discomfort leads to decreased activity, feeling lousy, and ultimately more pain. This is tragic because most back and neck pain is simple and easy to predict, prevent, or even reverse.

Life is not over because you were told that you have a bad back.

The good news is that back pain is not a standard symptom of getting older. It doesn't occur because we walk upright on two legs. It also doesn't happen because we lifted something wrong one day. However, bed rest and inactivity are more likely the culprits of the seemingly endless charade of back pain.

> "Every life properly lived is a beacon that others can follow."

For those of you who are athletic, you may have heard that abdominal crunches are great for treating the back. Beware! Unfortunately, abdominal exercises are not the answer for improving back pain. An imbalance may occur if your abdominal muscles are overworked or the only ones being worked. However, you don't need to stop exercising because someone told you that you shouldn't exercise due to a "bad back." Many people like me have actually found great relief with exercise.

Back and neck pain usually develop slowly over time without us even taking note. Just like any bad habit, it can cause trouble over time.

Sometimes, pain may come suddenly. It may occur after a car accident, a fall, or some other injury. However, the likelihood is that the pain was brewing beforehand from many simple bad habits. Rapid onset of the pain is like a heart attack developing over years that suddenly occurs with one more aggravating factor. The key is to identify and modify abusive patterns.

As previously mentioned, most of you are going to get the same diagnosis I got 10 years ago. You'll be told that you have to scale back on physical activity. Many of you may be sold on this lie.

I'm here to tell you that back pain is not the end. Don't stop doing what you love. Stay active. In fact, become more active! That's the answer to the diagnosis. That's the way to stay healthy and happy with a "bad back."

(If you've been diagnosed with arthritis, it's imperative that you receive a full medical clearance from your licensed physician before starting any exercise program. If you haven't read Step 9, please refer to it for establishing a correct exercise regimen.)

Warmly,

Francisco M. Torres, MD

Overcoming Pain with Healthy Practices

I've been an athlete all my life, as well as a highly competitive Certified Strength and Conditioning Specialist for athletes. For over 10 years, I have worked with weekend warriors, college athletes, and high level competitors. My line of work requires heavy lifting and maneuvering.

Severe back pain has plagued me almost half my life. Recently, I had to undergo emergency back surgery for sudden neurological deficits. Can you image a re-herniated lumbar disc splitting downwards into your spinal cord, shutting off sensory and motor nerve supply to your lower leg and foot? Well, that's what happened to me!

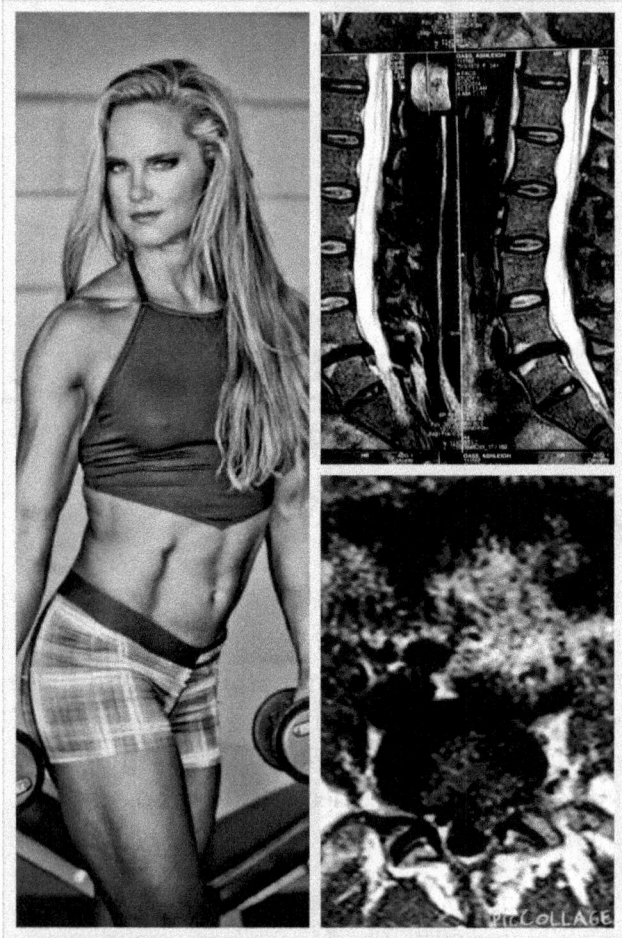

While some may have required extensive recovery time after undergoing such a surgery, it took only days for me to recover. In fact, I was able to return to the gym for training almost right away. A few months later, I even competed in a physique show. Performing in the show required strenuous exercise training which paid off in more ways than one. I placed second overall in my respective divisions, but my pain also improved greatly.

The difference between my recovery time and that of the average patient was due to several factors:

1. an excellent neurosurgeon (Dr. Chris Mickler)

2. retraining my back, including spinal training

3. a lifetime of health practices and nutritional strategies outlined in this book

Along with Dr. Torres, I too want to encourage you to keep moving. It's one of the best therapies to help you rehabilitate your back and improve pain, as well as arthritis symptoms.

Best Wishes!

Ashleigh Gass

Closing

We hope you've learned something in these pages. We have a passion for helping those who desire to live forever young. If you would like more information, please visit our website at www.ForeverYoung.MD.

If you've enjoyed our book, please leave feedback. It's only through your insights and support that we will have any success getting our passionate message out to many others. Our sincere contributions to health mean nothing without your support.

Thank you for reading. Keep thriving to the end!

Other Books You May Enjoy

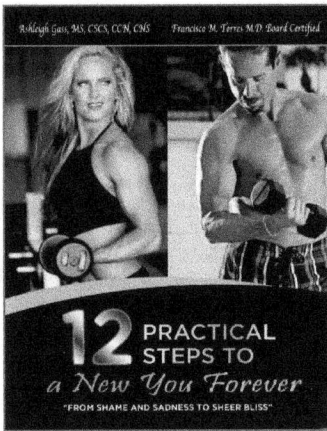

12 Practical Steps to a New You Forever – *From Shame and Sadness to Sheer Bliss*

by Dr. Franscisco M. Torres & Ashleigh Gass

One Size Does NOT Fit All Diet Plan – *Meal Planning That Will Boost Your Metabolism, Break Through Plateaus, and Help You Achieve Maximum Fat Loss Today!*

by Abby Campbell

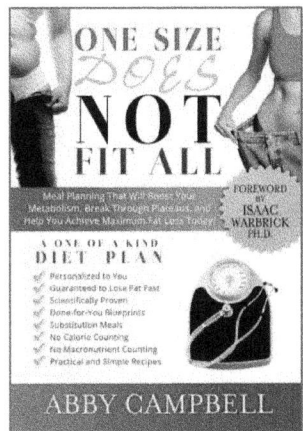

"Coaching is about inspiration – not direction."

~Dr. Torres

Endnotes

[1] National Center for Chronic Disease Prevention and Health Promotion | Division of Population Health. (2014, March 17). *Arthritis-Related Statistics*. Retrieved from http://www.cdc.gov/arthritis/data_statistics/arthritis_related_stats.htm.

[2] Ibid.

[3] Ibid.

[4] Ibid.

[5] Borestein, D. (2012, February). *Neck Pain.* Retrieved from https://www.rheumatology.org/Practice/Clinical/Patients/Diseases_And_Conditions/Neck_Pain/.

[6] Perlman, A., Sabina, A. & Williams, A. et al. (2006, December 11/25). Massage Therapy for Osteoarthritis of the Knee: A Randomized Controlled Trial. *JAMA Internal Medicine 166(22)*, 2533-2538. doi: 10.1001/archinte.166.22.2533. Retrieved from http://archinte.jamanetwork.com/article.aspx?articleid=769544.

[7] Bernstein, Susan. (2015, March 15). *Benefits of Massage.* Retrieved from http://www.arthritistoday.org/arthritis-treatment/natural-and-alternative-treatments/remedies-and-therapies/benefits-of-massage.php.

[8] Cherkin, D., Sherman, K. & Kahn, J., et al. (2011, July 5). A Comparison of the Effects of 2 Types of Massage and Usual Care on Chronic Low Back Pain:

A Randomized Controlled Trial. *Annals of Internal Medicine 155(1)*, 1-9. doi: 10.7326/0003-4819-155-1-201107050-00002. Retrieved from http://annals.org/article.aspx?articleid=747008.

9 Field, T., Diego, M. & Hernandez-Reif, M. (2010, May). Moderate Pressure is Essential for Massage Therapy Effects. *International Journal of Neuroscience 120(5)*, 381-385. doi: 10.3109/0020745093579475. Retrieved from http://informahealthcare.com/doi/abs/10.3109/00207450903579475.

10 Tam, L., Leung, P. & Li, T., et al. (2007, November 3). Acupuncture in the Treatment of Rheumatoid Arthritis: a Double-Blind Controlled Pilot Study. *BMC Complementary and Alternative Medicine 7(35)*. doi: 10.1186/1472-6882-7-35. Retrieved from http://www.biomedcentral.com/1472-6882/7/35.

11 Witt, C., Brinkhaus, B. & Reinhold, T., et al. (2006). Efficacy, Effectiveness, Safety and Costs of Acupuncture for Chronic Pain – Results of a Large Research Initiative. *Acupuncture in Medicine, 24(33)*, 33-39. doi: 10.1136/aim.24.Suppl.33. Retrieved from http://aim.bmj.com/content/24/supplement/33.abstract.

12 CDC/National Center for Health Statistics. (2015, January 14). *Obesity and Overweight*. Retrieved from http://www.cdc.gov/nchs/fastats/obesity-overweight.htm.

13 Pietrzykowska, N. (2015). *Benefits of 5-10 Percent Weight-loss*. Retrieved from http://www.obesityaction.org/educational-resources/resource-articles-2/general-articles/benefits-of-5-10-percent-weight-loss.

[14] Messier, S, Guetkunst, D. & Davis, C., et al. (2005, July). Weight Loss Reduces Knee-Joint Loads in Overweight and Obese Older Adults with Knee Osteoarthritis. *Arthritis and Rheumatism, 52(7)*, 2026-2032. doi: 10.1002/art.21139. Retrieve from http://www.ncbi.nlm.nih.gov/pubmed/15986358.

[15] Hoy, D., March, L & Brooks, P., et al. (2014, March 24). The Global Burden of Low Back Pain: Estimates from the Global Burden of Disease 2010 Study. *Annals of Rheumatic Disease, 73*, 968-974. doi: 10.1136/annrheumdis-2013-2014428. Retrieved from http://ard.bmj.com/content/73/6/968.full.

[16] Esser, S. & Bailey, A. (2011, December). Effects of Exercise and Physical Activity on Knee Arthritis. *Current Pain and Headache Reports, 15(6)*, 423-430. doi: 10.1007/s11916-011-0225-z. Retrieved from http://www.ncbi.nlm.nih.gov/pubmed/21956792.

[17] Peters, John, Wyatt, H. & Foster, G., et al. (2014, June). The Effects of Water and Non-Nutritive Sweetened Beverages on Weight Loss During a 12-Week Weight Loss Treatment Program. *Obesity, 22(6)*, 1415-1421. doi: 10.1002.oby.20737. Retrieved from http://anschutz.new-media-release.com/study/downloads/oby20737_NNS_study.pdf.

[18] Yang, Q. (2010, June). Gain Weight by "Going Diet?" Artificial Sweeteners and the Neurobiology of Sugar Cravings. *Yale Journal of Biology and Medicine, 83(2)*, 101-108. Retrieved from http://www.ncbi.nlm.nih.gov/pmc/articles/PMC2892765/.

[19] Wing, R. & Phelan, S. (2005, July). Long-Term Weight Loss Maintenance. *American Journal of*

Clinical Nutrition, 82(1), 222S-225S. Retrieved from
http://ajcn.nutrition.org/content/82/1/222S.long.

[20] Gass, M. (1996). *Heritage Writing*. Clackamas,
Oregon: Sieben Hill.

[21] West, J., Otte, C. & Gehe, K., et al. (2004,
October). Effects of Hatha Yoga and African Dance
on Perceived Stress, Affect, and Salivary Cortisol.
Annals of Behavioral Medicine, 28(2), 114-118.
Retrieved from
http://www.ncbi.nlm.nih.gov/pubmed/15454358.

[22] National Sleep Foundation. (2015). *How Much
Sleep Do We Really Need?* Retrieved from
http://sleepfoundation.org/how-sleep-works/how-
much-sleep-do-we-really-need?page=0%2C0.

[23] Heffron, T. (2014, March 10). *Insomnia
Awareness Day Facts and Stats*. Retrieved from
http://www.sleepeducation.com/news/2014/03/10/
insomnia-awareness-day-facts-and-stats.

[24] Simano, M., Haythorthwaite, J. & Smith, M.
(2012, April 26). *Change in Attitude May Ease
Chronic Pain by Aiding Sleep, Study Suggests*.
Retrieved by
http://www.hopkinsmedicine.org/news/media/rele
ases/change_in_attitude_may_ease_chronic_pain_
by_aiding_sleep_study_suggests.

[25] Irwin, M., Wang, M. & Campomayor, C., et al.
(2006, September 18). Sleep Deprivation and
Activation of Morning Levels of Cellular and
Genomic Markers of Inflammation. *JAMA Internal
Medicine, 166(16)*, 1756-1762. doi
10.1001/archinte.166.16.1756. Retrieved from
http://archinte.jamanetwork.com/article.aspx?articl
eid=410868.

[26] Riskowski, J., Dufour, A. & Hannan, M. (2011, July 11). Arthritis, Foot Pain & Shoe Wear: Current Musculoskeletal Research on Feet. *Current Opinion in Rheumatology, 23(2)*, 148-155. doi 10.1097/BOR.0b013e3283422cf5. Retrieved from http://www.ncbi.nlm.nih.gov/pmc/articles/PMC313 2870/.

[27] Hawke, F., Burns, J. & Radford, et al. (2008, July 16). Custom-Made Foot Orthoses for the Treatment of Foot Pain. *The Cochrane Collaboration®*. doi: 10.1002/14651858.CD006801.pub2. Retrieved from http://onlinelibrary.wiley.com/doi/10.1002/146518 58.CD006801.pub2/full.

[28] Giordullo, S. (2014, September 14). *Tread Wisely When Choose Orthotics*. Retrieved from http://www.angieslist.com/articles/tread-wisely-when-choosing-orthotics.htm.

[29] Riegler, H. (1987, May). Orthotic Devices for the Foot. *Orthopedic Reviews, 16(5)*, 293-303. Retrieved from http://www.ncbi.nlm.nih.gov/pubmed/3454941.

[30] Bransby-Zachary, M., Stother, I. & Wilkinson, R. (1990, July). Peak Pressures in the Forefoot. *Journal of Bone and Joint Surgery, 72(4)*, 718-721. Retrieved from http://www.bjj.boneandjoint.org.uk/content/72-B/4/718.long.

[31] Bartlett, S. (2011, October 13). *Role of Exercise in Arthritis Management*. Retrieved from http://www.hopkinsarthritis.org/patient-corner/disease-management/role-of-exercise-in-arthritis-management/#ref 2.

[32] American College of Sports Medicine. (1997). *ACSM's Exercise Management for Persons with*

Chronic Diseases and Disabilities. Champaign, Illinois: Human Kinetics, 1997.

33 Ettinger, W., Burns, R. & Messier, S., et al. (1997, January). A Randomized Trial Comparing Aerobic Exercise and Resistance Exercise with a Health Education Program in Older Adults with Knee Osteoarthritis: The Fitness Arthritis and Seniors Trial (FAST). *The Journal of the American Medical Association, 277(1)*, 25-31. doi: 10.1001/jama.1997.03540250033028. Retrieve from http://jama.jamanetwork.com/article.aspx?articleid =412600.

34 Anderson, R., Blair, S. & Cheskin, L., et al. (1997, September 1). Encouraging Patients to Become More Physically Active: The Physician's Role. *Annals of Internal Medicine, 127(5)*, 395-400. doi: 10.7326/0003-4819-127-5-199709010-00010. Retrieved from http://annals.org/article.aspx?articleid=710792.

35 Minor, M., Hewett, J. & Webel, R. (1989, November). Efficacy of Physical Conditioning Exercise in Patients with Rheumatoid Arthritis and Osteoarthritis. *Arthritis Rheumatology, 32(11)*, 1396-1405. doi: 10.1002/anr.1780321108. Retrieved from http://onlinelibrary.wiley.com/doi/10.1002/anr.178 0321108/abstract.

36 The President's Council on Physical Fitness and Sports. (1999, November 17). *Physical Activity and Health: A Report of the Surgeon General*. Retrieved from http://www.cdc.gov/nccdphp/sgr/olderad.htm.

37 American College of Sports Medicine. (1997). ACSM's Exercise Management for Persons with

Chronic Diseases and Disabilities. Champaign, Illinois: Human Kinetics, 1997.

[38] Wang, X., Kou, X. & Mao, J., et al. (2012, May 9). Sustained Inflammation Induces Degeneration of the Temporomandibular Joint. *Journal of Dental Research, 91(5),* 499-505. doi: 10.1177/0022034512441946. Retrieved from http://www.ncbi.nlm.nih.gov/pmc/articles/PMC33 27731/#__ffn__sectitle,

[39] Hedbom, E. & Hauselmann, H. (2002, January). Molecular Aspects of Pathogenesis in Osteoarthritis: The Role of Inflammation. *Cellular and Molecular Life Sciences, 59(1),* 45-53. Retrieved from http://www.ncbi.nlm.nih.gov/pubmed/11846032.

[40] de Git, K. & Adan, R. (2015, March). Leptin Resistance in Diet-Induced Obesity: The Role of Hypothalamic Inflammation. *Obesity Reviews, 16(3),* 207-224. doi: 10.1111/obr.12243. Retrieved from http://onlinelibrary.wiley.com/doi/10.1111/obr.1224 3/full.

[41] Lorente-Cebrian, S., Costa, A. & Navas-Carretero, S. (2015, March 11). An Update on the Role of Omega-3 Fatty Acids on Inflammatory and Degenerative Diseases. *Journal of Physiology and Biochemistry.* doi: 10.1007/s13105-015-0395-y. Retrieved from http://onlinelibrary.wiley.com/doi/10.1111/obr.1224 3/full.

[42] Vyaskh, A., Ratheesh, M. & Rajmohanan, T., et al. (2014, May 2014). Polyphenolics Isolated From Virgin Coconut Oil Inhibits Adjuvant Induced Arthritis in Rats Through Antioxidant and Anti-Inflammatory Action. *International Immunopharmacology, 20(1),* 124-130. doi: 10.1016/j.intimp.2014.02.026. Retrieved from

http://www.sciencedirect.com/science/article/pii/S
1567576914000800.

43 Musumeci, G., Frovato, F & Pichier, K. (2013,
December). Extra-Virgin Olive Oil Diet and Mild
Physical Activity Prevent Cartilage Degeneration in
an Osteoarthritis Model: An In Vivo and In Vitro
Study on Lubricin Expression. *The Journal of
Nutritional Biochemistry, 24(12)*, 2064-2075.
Retrieved from
http://www.ncbi.nlm.nih.gov/pubmed/24369033.

44 Boeing, H., Bechthold, A. & Bub, A., et al. (2012,
September). Critical Review: Vegetables and Fruit in
the Prevention of Chronic Diseases. *European
Journal of Nutrition, 51(6)*, 637-663. doi:
10.1007/s00394-012-0380-y. Retrieved from
http://www.ncbi.nlm.nih.gov/pmc/articles/PMC341
9346/#Abs1title.

45 Tsau, J., Liu, H. & Chen, Y. (2010). Suppression of
Inflammatory Mediators by Cruciferous Vegetable-
Derived Indol-3-Carbinol and Phylethyl
Isothiocyanate in Lipopolysaccharide-Activated
Macrophages. *Mediators of Inflammation*. doi:
10.1155/2010/293642. Retrieved from
http://www.ncbi.nlm.nih.gov/pmc/articles/PMC28
55117/.

46 Vitetta, L. Coulson, S. & Linnane, A., et al. (2013,
December 2). The Gastrointestinal Micobiome and
Musculoskeletal Diseases: A Beneficial Role for
Probiotics and Prebiotics. *Pathogens, 2(4)*, 606-626.
doi: 10.3390/pathogens2040606. Retrieved from
http://www.ncbi.nlm.nih.gov/pmc/articles/PMC42
35701/.

47 Geng, Y., Zhu, S. & Lu, Z., et al. (2014). Anti-
Inflammatory Activity of Mycelial Extracts from
Medicinal Mushrooms. *International Journal of*

Medicinal Mushrooms, 16(4), 319-325. doi: 10.1615/IntJMushrooms. Retrieved from http://www.dl.begellhouse.com/journals/708ae68d 64b17c52,4c99b516238143af,0b6528d9687446ed.ht ml.

[48] Quintero-Fabian, S., Ortuno-Sahgun, D. & Vazquez-Carrera, M., et al. (2013, December 26). Alliin, A Garlic (Allium Satvum) Compound, Prevents LPS-Induced Inflammation in 3T3-L1 Adipocytes. *Mediators of Inflammation*. doi: 10.1155/2013/381815. Retrieved from http://www.ncbi.nlm.nih.gov/pmc/articles/PMC38 88727/.

[49] Joseph, S., Edirisingh, I. & Burton-Freeman, B. (2014, February 11). Berries: Anti-Inflammatory Effects in Humans. *Journal of Agricultural and Food Chemistry, 62(18)*, 3886-3903. Retrieved from http://pubs.acs.org/doi/pdfplus/10.1021/jf4044056 .

[50] Maroon, J., Bost, J. & Maroon, A. (2010). Natural Anti-Inflammatory Agents for Pain Relief. *Surgical Neurology International, 1(80)*. doi: 10.4103/2152-7806.73804. Retrieved from http://www.ncbi.nlm.nih.gov/pmc/articles/PMC301 1108/,

[51] Weiss, D. & Anderton, C. (2003, September 5). Determination of Catechins in Matcha Green Tea by Micellar Electrokinetic Chromatography. *Journal of Chromatography A, 1011(1-2)*, 173-180. Retrieved from http://www.ncbi.nlm.nih.gov/pubmed/14518774.

[52] Sengupta, K., Kolla, J. & Krishnaraju, A., et al. (2011, August). Cellular and Molecular Mechanisms of Anti-Inflammatory Effect of Aflapin: A Novel Boswellia Serrata Extract. *Molecular and Cellular*

Biochemistry, 354(1-2), 189-197. doi:
10.1007/s11010-011-0818-1. Retrieved from
http://www.ncbi.nlm.nih.gov/pubmed/21479939.

[53] Henrotin, Y., Marty, M. & Mobasheri, A. (2014,
July). What is the Current Status of Chondroitin
Sulfate and Glucosamine for the Treatment of Knee
Osteoarthritis? *Maturitas, 78(3)*, 184-187. doi:
10.1016/j.maturitas.2014.04.015. Retrieved from
http://www.maturitas.org/article/S0378-
5122(14)00134-0/abstract.

[54] Jerosch, J. (2011, August 2). Effects of
Glucosamine and Chondroitin Sulfate on Cartilage
Metabolism in OA: Outlook on Other Nutrient
Partners Especially Omega-3 Fatty Acids.
International Journal of Rheumatology. doi:
10.1155/2011/969012. Retrieved from
http://www.ncbi.nlm.nih.gov/pmc/articles/PMC315
0191/.

[55] Cameron, M., Gagnier, J. & Chrubasik, S. (2011,
February 16). Herbal Therapy for Treating
Rheumatoid Arthritis. *Cochrane Database of
Systematic Reviews*. doi:
10.1002/14651858.CD002948.pub2. Retrieved from
http://onlinelibrary.wiley.com/enhanced/doi/10.10
02/14651858.CD002948.pub2.

[56] Therkleson, T. (2014, January 29). Ginger Therapy
for Osteoarthritis: A Typical Case. *Journal of
Holistic Nursing, 32*, 232-239. doi
10.1177/0898010113520467. Retrieved from
http://jhn.sagepub.com/content/32/3/232.long.

[57] Gurenwald, J., Petzold, E. & Busch, R., et al.
(2009, September). Effect of Glucosamine Sulfate
with or without Omega-3 Fatty Acids in Patients
with Osteoarthritis. *Advances in Therapy, 26(9)*,
858-871. doi: 10.1007/s12325-009-0060-3.

Retrieved from
http://link.springer.com/article/10.1007%2Fs12325
-009-0060-3.

58 Cho, S., Jung, Y. & Seong, S. (2003, June). Clinical
Efficacy and Safety of Lyprinol, a Patented Extract
from Nw Zealand Green-Lipped Mussel (Perna
Canaliculus) in Patients with Osteoarthritis of the
Hip and Knee: A Multicenter 2-Month Clinical Trial.
*European Annals of Allergy and Clinical
Immunology, 35(6)*, 212-216. Retrieved from
http://www.ncbi.nlm.nih.gov/pubmed/12872680.

59 Zawadzki, M. Janosch, C. & Szechinski, J. (2013,
June 5). Perna Canaliculus Lipid Complex PCSO-
520™ Demonstrated Pain Relief for Osteoarthritis
Patients Benchmarked Against Fish Oil, a
Randomized Trial without Placebo Control. *Marine
Drugs, 11(6)*, 1920-1935. doi: 10.3390/mc11061920.
Retrieved from
http://www.ncbi.nlm.nih.gov/pmc/articles/PMC372
1214/#__ffn_sectitle.

60 Tashiro, T., Seino, S. & Sato, T. (2012, October 16).
Oral Administration of Polymer Hyaluronic Acid
Alleviates Symptoms of Knee Osteoarthritis: A
Double-Blind, Placebo-Controlled Study Over a 12-
Month Period. *The Scientific World Journal*. doi:
10.1100/2012/167928. Retrieved from
http://www.hindawi.com/journals/tswj/2012/16792
8/.

61 Christen, W., Schaumber, D. & Glynn, R., et al.
(2011, June). Dietary w-3 Fatty Acid and Fish Intake
and Incident Age-Related Macular Degeneration in
Women. *JAMA Ophthalmology, 129(7)*, 921-929. doi
10.1001/archophthalmol.2011.34. Retrieved from
http://archopht.jamanetwork.com/article.aspx?artic
leid=1106372.

[62] Cisar, P., Jany, R. & Waczulikova, I., et al. (2008, August). Effect of Pine Bark Extract (Pycogenol) on Symptoms of Knee Osteoarthritis. *Phytotherapy Research, 22(8)*, 1087-1092. doi: 10.1002/ptr.2461. Retrieved from http://onlinelibrary.wiley.com/doi/10.1002/ptr.2461/abstract.

[63] Funk, J., Oyarzo, J. & Frye, J. (2006, March). Turmeric Extracts Containing Curcuminoids Prevent Experimental Rheumatoid Arthritis. *Journal of Natural Products, 69(3)*, 351-355. doi: 10.1021/np050327j. Retrieved from http://onlinelibrary.wiley.com/doi/10.1002/ptr.2461/abstracthttp://www.ncbi.nlm.nih.gov/pmc/articles/PMC2533857/pdf/nihms62829.pdf.

[64] Lal, B., Kapoor, A. & Asthana, O., et al. (1999, June). Efficacy of Curcumin in the Management of Chronic Anterior Uveitis. *Phytotherapy Research, 13(4)*, 318-322. Retrieved from http://www.ncbi.nlm.nih.gov/pubmed/10404539.

[65] Chandran, B. & Ajay Goel. (2012). A Randomized, Pilot Study to Assess the Efficacy and Safety of Curcumin in Patients with Active Rheumatoid Arthritis. *Phytotherapy Research.* doi: 10.1002/ptr.4639. Retrieved from http://www.equinenutriceuticals.com/pdf/RA-Study-BCM-95.pdf.

[66] Linetsky, F. & Willard, Fl. (1999, August). Regenerative Injection Therapy for Low Back Pain. *The Pain Clinic, 1(1), 19-23.*

[67] Tollison, C., Satterthwaite, J. & Tollison, J. (2002, January 15). Spinal Disc Disease. *Practical Pain Management* (pp. 411-430). Philadelphia, Pennsylvania: Lippincott Williams & Wilkins.

[68] Vora, A., Borg-Stein, J. & Nguyen, R. (2012, May). Regenerative Injection Therapy for Osteoarthritis: Fundamental Concepts and Evidence-Based Review. *PM&R, 4(5),* S104-S109. doi: 10.1016/j.pmri.2012.02.005. Retrieved from http://www.pmrjournal.org/article/S1934-1482(12)00070-6/abstract.

[69] Dumais, R., Benoit, C. & Dumais, A., et al. (2012, July 3). Effect of Regenerative Injection Therapy on Function and Pain in Patients with Knee Osteoarthritis: A Randomized Crossover Study. *Pain Medicine, 13(8),* 990-999. doi: 10.1111/j.1526-4637.2012.01422x. Retrieved from http://onlinelibrary.wiley.com/doi/10.1111/j.1526-4637.2012.01422.x/abstract.

[70] Topol, G. & Reeves, K. (2008, November). Regenerative Injection of Elite Athletes with Career-Altering Chronic Groin Pain Who Fail Conservative Treatment: A Consecutive Case Series. *American Journal of Physical Medicine & Rehabilitation, 87(11),* 890-902. doi: 10.1097/PHM.0b013e31818377b6. Retrieved from http://journals.lww.com/ajpmr/pages/articleviewer.aspx?year=2008&issue=11000&article=00004&type=abstract.

[71] Xia, Q., Zhu, S. & Wu, Y., et al. (2015, March 30). Intra-Articular Transplantation of Atsttrin-Transduced Mesenchymal Stem Cells Ameliorate Osteoarthritis Development. *Stem Cells Translational Medicine®.* doi: 10.5966/sctm.2014-0200. Retrieved from http://stemcellstm.alphamedpress.org/content/early/2015/03/29/sctm.2014-0200.long.

[72] Vega, A., Martin-Ferrero, M. & Del Canto, F., et al. (2015, March 27). Treatment of Knee Osteoarthritis with Allogeneic Bone Marrow Mesenchymal Stem

Cells: A Randomized Controlled Trial. *Transplantation*. Retrieved from http://www.ncbi.nlm.nih.gov/pubmed/25822648.

73 Su, C., Hsu, C. & Tsai, C., et al. (2015, March 31). Resistin Promotes Angiogenesis in Endothelial Progenitor Cells Through Inhibition of MicroRNA206: Potential Implications for Rheumatoid Arthritis. *Stem Cells*. doi: 10.1002/stem.2024. Retrieved from http://onlinelibrary.wiley.com/doi/10.1002/stem.2024/abstract.

74 Hu, J., Li, H. & Chi, G., et al. (2015, Jan 15). IL-1RA Gene-Transfected Bone Marrow-Derived Mesenchymal Stem Cells in APA Microcapsules Could Alleviate Rheumatoid Arthritis. *International Journal of Clinical and Experimental Medicine, 8(1)*, 706-713. Retrieved from http://www.ncbi.nlm.nih.gov/pmc/articles/PMC4358502/#__ffn_sectitle.

75 Liu, H., Ding, J. & Wang, J. (2015, March 16). Remission of Collagen-Induced Arthritis through Combination Therapy of Microfracture and Transplantation of Thermogel-Encapsulated Bone Marrow Mesenchymal Stem Cells. *PLoS ONE, 10(3)*, doi: 10.1371/journal.pone.0120596. Retrieved from http://www.ncbi.nlm.nih.gov/pmc/articles/PMC4361318/.

76 Xie, X., Zhang, C. & Tuan, R. (2014, February 25). Biology of Platelet-Rich Plasma and Its Clinical Application in Cartilage Repair. *Arthritis Research & Therapy, 16(1)*, 204. Retrieved from http://www.ncbi.nlm.nih.gov/pmc/articles/PMC3978832/.

77 Raeissadat, S., Rayagani, S. & Hassanabadi, H., et al. (2015, January 7). Knee Osteoarthritis Injection

Choices: Platelet-Rich Plasma (PRP) Versus Hyaluronic Acid (A One-Year Randomized Clinical Trial). *Clinical Medicine Insights, Arthritis and Musculoskeletal Disorders, 8*, 1-8. doi: 10.4137/CMAMD.S17894. Retrieved from http://www.ncbi.nlm.nih.gov/pmc/articles/PMC42 87055/.

[78] Rayegani, S., Raeissadat, S. & Teheri, M., et al. (2014, September 18). Does Intra Articular Platelet Rich Plasma Injection Improve Function, Pain and Quality of Life in Patients with Osteoarthritis of the Knee? A Randomized Clinical Trial. *Orthopedic Reviews, 6(3)*, 5405. doi: 10.4081/or.2014.5405. Retrieved from http://www.ncbi.nlm.nih.gov/pmc/articles/PMC419 5987/.

www.ingramcontent.com/pod-product-compliance
Lightning Source LLC
Chambersburg PA
CBHW050121280326
41933CB00010B/1190